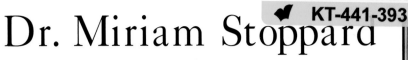
Dr. Miriam Stoppard
HEALTHY PREGNANCY

HEALTHCARE

DORLING KINDERSLEY
London • New York • Sydney • Moscow

A DORLING KINDERSLEY BOOK

DESIGN AND EDITORIAL Edward Kinsey and Jaqueline Jackson

SENIOR MANAGING ART EDITOR Lynne Brown
MANAGING EDITOR Jemima Dunne

SENIOR ART EDITOR Karen Ward
SENIOR EDITOR Penny Warren

PRODUCTION Antony Heller

First published in Great Britain in 1998 by
Dorling Kindersley Limited, 9 Henrietta Street,
Covent Garden, London WC2E 8PS

Visit us on the World Wide Web at http://www.dk.com

A CIP catalogue record for this book is available
from the British Library

ISBN 0-7513-0551-0

Reproduced by Colourscan, Singapore and IGS, Radstock, Avon
Printed in Hong Kong by Wing King Tong

HEALTHY
PREGNANCY

CONTENTS

INTRODUCTION 6

INTRODUCTION

When you discover you are pregnant, your excitement will probably be tinged with apprehension. This isn't surprising when you consider the enormous changes that go on in a woman's body to nurture her unborn baby from conception to birth. Pregnancy is not an illness, it's a normal part of human life, but it's sensible to do all you can to maintain your own and your baby's health, and to prepare yourself for labour, birth and the care of your baby afterwards.

PREPARATION FOR BIRTH

Pregnancy and labour place heavy demands on your body, so preparing yourself is important. While there is no special diet for pregnancy, choose a balanced diet with plenty of fruit and vegetables to give you the nutrients you need. There's no need to "eat for two", but eating sensibly and not skimping on meals are important, especially if you are working. It's sensible to exercise regularly as well because not only will you be able to cope better with the extra weight of pregnancy, but you may find labour easier if your muscles are in tone. Learning how to relax and to control the pain of contractions through breathing are also beneficial. The forty weeks of pregnancy give you time to establish a bond with your unborn baby. Communicate with your baby by stroking your abdomen and responding to fetal movements with talking or singing.

A SENSUAL PREGNANCY

You may find your relationship with your partner is enhanced; due to high levels of hormones, many women find they are capable of greater sexual arousal during pregnancy. Provided that you feel comfortable (your increasing size may make some positions difficult) and your partner is sensitive, you may find this a time of renewed intimacy as you approach your new status as parents.

BECOMING A PARENT

Having a baby is one of the most important events in our lives and, ideally, it should be planned with care. Preparing for parenthood will help you negotiate the demands of pregnancy and childbirth with confidence. This is also a time to reassess your life, because parenthood will have a fundamental effect on all aspects of it. You owe it to your child to prepare for pregnancy by changing to a more healthy lifestyle because a baby's health depends to a large extent on the diet and lifestyle of his parents at conception: whether you smoke, drink or take drugs; how fit you are and how well you eat are of paramount importance.

FIT FOR PARENTHOOD

A successful pregnancy and labour, and the birth of a healthy baby, are the responsibilities of both parents to an equal degree. A baby's health depends to a large extent on the health of her parents at the moment of conception, and her well-being can be affected not only by long-standing medical conditions or familial genetic defects, but also by her parents' lifestyle before conception. Many couples do not plan for pregnancy with the same care as they plan for other significant life events, yet it is one of the most important things you can do. Starting a family needs a time of reassessment because becoming a parent will fundamentally change your life.

LIFESTYLE CONSIDERATIONS

Many things that we take for granted – who we are and what we do – will affect or be affected by having a baby.

Time Most young people are extremely busy and many new parents assume that their baby will somehow fit in. They don't. Babies and children need a lot of time and attention, and parents will always have less time than they did before – for themselves, for each other and for other people.

Costs The average experience is that you will spend 15–25 percent of your income, regardless of how much you earn or the size of your family, on child-related expenses such as clothing and equipment. But there are also hidden costs such as heating and transportation as well as what you may give up for your children – meals out, holidays and, perhaps, some of your ambitions.

Relationships It is not only your relationship with your partner that changes when you have a baby. Your relationship with your parents also changes, and you may find that you grow away from your childless friends as you enjoy friendships with other new parents.

Smoking This is one of the most damaging factors to the health of your unborn baby and the major cause of avoidable health problems. The associated risks include

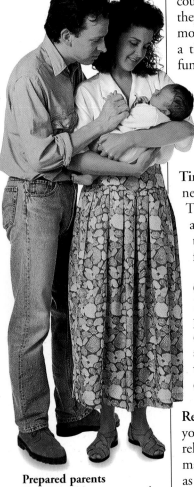

Prepared parents
Happy, healthy parents make happy, healthy babies, so make sure you are fit for parenthood before you start trying for a baby.

miscarriage and stillbirth, damage to the placenta, a low birthweight baby that fails to thrive, and an increased chance of fetal abnormalities. A man who continues to smoke while his partner is pregnant risks damaging the health of his unborn baby through passive smoking. It can also have long-term effects – children of heavy smokers tested at five, seven and 11 years have been found to suffer from impaired growth and learning difficulties.

Alcohol This is a poison that may damage the sperm and ovum before conception, as well as the developing embryo. The main risks to the unborn baby are mental retardation, retarded growth and damage to the brain and nervous system – well documented as fetal alcohol syndrome. Alcohol can also cause stillbirth.
Research suggests that the effect of alcohol is variable: some heavy drinkers seem to get away with it, while other women who drink only a small amount don't. The only certainty is that there is no effect if alcohol is avoided.

Drugs Over-the-counter medicines should only be taken when necessary, and street drugs should definitely be cut out before you conceive. Marijuana interferes with the normal production of male sperm, and the effects take three to nine months to wear off. Hard drugs such as cocaine, heroin and morphine can damage the chromosomes, leading to fetal abnormalities and addictions.

Age If you delay pregnancy until your 30s, and even 40s, this is no more hazardous as long as you are fit and healthy. However, some problems such as chromosomal defects, for example Down's syndrome (see p. 12), occur more frequently with the increasing age of both parents.

Hazards Be aware of your environment, both in and out of the home, and avoid anything that is potentially dangerous. What we eat, where we work and sometimes who we meet may be risky for a pregnant woman (see p. 56).

Diet and exercise Both are vital to your health and the health of your baby. You need to eat a balanced diet with plenty of raw fruit and vegetables (see pp. 22–27), coupled with moderate exercise (see pp. 32–39) because the fitter you are, the better your body will cope with labour.

STOPPING CONTRACEPTION

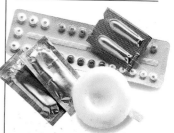

Barrier methods, such as the diaphragm and sheath, can be dispensed with straight away. However, if you are on the pill or are using an IUD, you need to plan ahead.

The pill It is advisable to stop taking the pill a month before trying to conceive, so that you have at least one normal menstrual period before becoming pregnant. However, there is some evidence to suggest that women are more fertile immediately after stopping the pill, so this could be the ideal time to try if you have had problems conceiving.

If you think that you are pregnant while taking the pill, consult your doctor at once. Some forms of the pill contain a high dose of progestogen (synthetic progesterone) that may interfere with early fetal development.

The intrauterine device Most IUDs, or coils, work by irritating the lining of the uterus so that the fertilized egg cannot implant. Some IUDs also contain progesterone, which could harm the fetus. It is best to have any IUD removed before becoming pregnant.

URINE TESTS

If sugar is found in your urine it may mean you have diabetes or, as is more likely, that some sugar has leaked through your kidneys, whose threshold to sugar is lowered by your pregnant state. Further tests will be necessary to make sure.

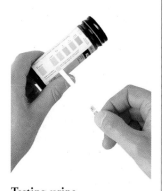

Testing urine
A chemically impregnated strip is dipped into a sample of your urine. The colour it turns to indicates if sugar is present when the strip is compared with a chart that shows glucose levels.

HEALTH CONSIDERATIONS

If you have a chronic long-term condition, such as diabetes mellitus, heart disease or epilepsy, you should not be discouraged from having children. However, you must talk things over with your doctor before becoming pregnant, so that your pregnancy can be managed effectively and in certain situations your medication changed.

Asthma This is usually controlled by inhalation of bronchodilator drugs and inhaled steroids. There seems to be little risk to the growing fetus from the medication, as long as steroids are inhaled properly, although sometimes labour may be brought on prematurely.

If you are asthmatic, you need to be extra careful throughout pregnancy because stress and tension, as well as dust, pollen and pollution, can cause an attack, which may increase the chances of a miscarriage. Stress is a trigger, so rest well and try some relaxation exercises.

Epilepsy Research has found that pregnancy has a variable effect on the frequency and intensity of fits, with 50 percent of epileptic mothers unaffected, 40 percent slightly improved, and 10 percent made worse.

Drug treatment must be continued during pregnancy, but you will need to be seen frequently by your doctor who can adjust your drug dosage. If you take phenytoin, absorption of folic acid can be affected and folic acid supplements are always given to prevent damage to the fetus. Most pregnant women can change to sodium valproate, which does not have the same effect. If you suffer from epilepsy, discuss this with your doctor well before you hope to conceive.

Diabetes mellitus When the pancreas produces insufficient insulin to cope with glucose (sugar) levels in the body, diabetes results. Pregnancy hormones have an anti-insulin effect, which increases the severity of established diabetes, and can also lead to the development of gestational diabetes in those with an underlying tendency. The urine of all mothers-to-be is routinely screened for sugar and ketones (the usual indicator of diabetes), and any woman with a family background of diabetes ought to be tested before attempting to conceive.

Insulin-dependent diabetics must monitor their blood-sugar levels extremely closely, since diabetes can lead to very large babies and fetal abnormalities such as heart and respiratory problems, as well as maternal complications. However, with strict control, every diabetic mother has an excellent chance of having a healthy baby.

Heart disease Women with a diagnosed condition will be given specialized advice according to its nature. However, as a general rule, it is advisable to avoid over-activity – try to rest each afternoon for at least two hours, and spend ten hours in bed at night.

The majority of women with heart disease have easy, spontaneous labours. During labour the additional strain on the heart is intermittent and, in total, is less than that imposed upon the heart in the third trimester.

Kidney disease A pregnant woman with kidney disease must be carefully monitored, and as long as the kidneys remove waste effectively, pregnancy can continue, but if there is poor fetal growth, early induction of labour will be recommended. (Renal dialysis does pose a risk because the mother's kidneys are unlikely to be able to cope with the additional waste from the fetus.)

Sexually transmitted disease Herpes is only a risk to your baby if you have your first outbreak in the last quarter of your pregnancy and you have symptoms at the time of your baby's birth. A herpes simplex II virus infection may lead to growth retardation in your baby. If you have no symptoms, and are not shedding the virus from sores in your cervix or vagina, the risk that your baby will become infected is less than one per thousand.

AIDS Infected women who become pregnant have a high risk of transmitting the virus to their babies either during birth, or by breastfeeding. To reduce the chances, mothers are treated in a special clinic where the severity of their condition is assessed. They are now given antiviral drugs during pregnancy, advised to have the baby by Caesarean section and not to breastfeed. The baby will not necessarily be born infected, but it can't be confirmed immediately whether the baby has the disease since it takes 18 months for the mother's antibodies to clear the baby's system.

RUBELLA

If you are considering pregnancy, before trying to conceive, ask your doctor or the hospital to give you a test to see if you have antibodies to the rubella (German measles) virus.

Don't assume you are immune to the disease if you have been vaccinated in the past – the antibodies lose their efficiency after a period of time, so check. If you are not immune, you should be vaccinated. However, after a successful vaccination, you should wait at least three months before you try to conceive, as the vaccine is live.

If you come into contact with someone who has, or is suspected of having, rubella, tell your doctor immediately, and a blood sample will be taken and sent to a laboratory for antibody testing.

Depending on the result, the test may be repeated in ten days. Should this test suggest that you have rubella, you and your partner will have to face the decision of whether to abort the pregnancy at this point. Some doctors recommend giving antibodies in the form of gamma globulin to help avoid fetal damage.

TAKE CARE

Rubella, particularly if caught in the first three months of pregnancy, can cause malformations in your baby. These may include deafness, blindness and heart disease.

DOWN'S SYNDROME

This chromosomal disorder occurs when the fertilized egg has 47 chromosomes instead of the usual 46.

In most cases, the egg itself is defective, being formed with the extra chromosome, or the sperm may be similarly affected. This type of Down's syndrome is known as trisomy. Or one parent may have a chromosomal abnormality that results in the child inheriting extra chromosomal material. This is known as translocation. Down's syndrome is diagnosed by chorionic villus sampling or amniocentesis.

The risk of having a Down's syndrome baby increases in women over the age of 35 but can also be caused by an older father.

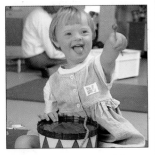

Down's syndrome child
One baby in every 1,000 will be born with this disorder. Down's syndrome is the result of trisomy, which is random, or translocation, which is inherited. It is therefore vital to determine the cause of any family history of Down's syndrome.

GENETIC CONSIDERATIONS

Within the nucleus of each cell are genes and chromosomes that contain DNA, which determines the growth and functioning of the body (see also p. 14). Genetic disorders occur when genes and chromosomes are abnormal. There are three reasons why genetic diseases can occur: a single gene may be defective, there may be a fault in the number or shape of chromosomes, or several genes may be faulty. There may also be complicating environmental factors. A single gene that is defective and results in a genetic disorder can be either dominant or recessive, a mutation, or attached to the X chromosome (see column, right). Abnormal chromosomes that result in genetic disorders are usually new mutations, although they can sometimes be inherited.

Where more than one gene or environmental factor is involved in producing a disorder, there is as yet no straightforward method of determining why it has happened. If either partner has a history of a genetic disease or condition in their extended family, counselling (see p. 16) should be sought. The number of reliable tests for genetic diseases that can be performed is increasing yearly, although they cannot predict the severity of the condition. The ultimate decision about whether to attempt to conceive, to go ahead with an existing pregnancy, or to request a termination will always rest with you, the parents. Bear in mind, however, that although a handicapped child will need special care, many such children are both affectionate and responsive, and can lead happy, fulfilled lives.

DOMINANT GENETIC DISEASES

Fatal diseases caused by dominant genes are rare because affected individuals normally die before they can pass on the genes. However, some conditions, such as familial hypercholesterolaemia (see below) are manageable.

Familial hypercholesterolaemia (FH) This is the most common dominant genetic disease. With FH the blood cholesterol levels are so high that there is a risk of heart attacks and other complications caused by narrowing of the arteries. The condition can be detected at birth by a test in which a sample of the baby's blood is taken.

RECESSIVE GENETIC DISEASES

A defective recessive gene is usually masked by a normal dominant one. However, if both parents carry a defective recessive gene, each of their children has a one in four chance of inheriting both recessive genes (and therefore one of several disorders) or neither, and a two in four chance of being a carrier. Thus there are always more people who are carriers rather than sufferers.

Cystic fibrosis CF is the most common recessive gene disorder. One in 20 of the Caucasian population carries the CF gene, and one in 2,000 Caucasian babies born is affected by the disease. In non-Caucasians, the incidence is about one in 90,000. This disease mainly affects the lungs and the digestive system. The mucus in the lungs becomes thick and sticky and accumulates, causing chest infections. The mucus also blocks the ducts of various organs, particularly the pancreas, thus preventing the normal flow of digestive enzymes. If not treated promptly, CF results in malnutrition. Over 60 percent of sufferers survive into adulthood, although few are in good health.

Sickle-cell anaemia This is the most common genetic disease among black people (one in 400). It is so called because the red cells are sickle-shaped from defective haemoglobin; this causes the red cells to break down and the small blood vessels to clog, which may result in a stroke. It is usually diagnosed by a blood test. Sufferers are susceptible to meningitis and other serious infections.

Thalassaemia This is common among Asians, blacks, and people of Mediterranean descent. It produces anaemia and chronic ill health, and blood transfusions may sometimes be necessary. A blood test will reveal the disease and other tests will indicate if the haemoglobin level is reduced. Not all cases are severe.

Tay-Sach's disease Common among Ashkenazic Jews, this is a fatal condition resulting in deterioration of the brain caused by deficiency in enzymes. Few children with the disease live beyond three years, and no adequate treatment is known. Tay-Sach's is diagnosed by testing blood for enzyme deficiency.

GENDER-LINKED DISEASES

These are conditions caused by defects on the X chromosome. If a second normal X chromosome is present, as in a healthy female, the defect won't show because it is masked. Women therefore carry the disease. If, however, a Y chromosome is present, as in a male, the disease will express itself, as a Y chromosome can't mask an X chromosome. Therefore males are affected.

Haemophilia This happens when the crucial clotting factor VIII is missing and results in profuse bleeding from any injury, external or internal. Effective treatment with factor VIII derived from normal blood is now available to haemophiliacs, and they can lead relatively normal lives. Diagnosis can be made from a sample of fetal blood at 18–20 weeks of pregnancy.

***Duchenne muscular dystrophy** This is the most common type of muscular dystrophy and affects only boys (one per 5,000). Between the ages of four and ten, a boy with Duchenne muscular dystrophy will lose his ability to walk, and is usually confined to a wheelchair during his comparatively short life. The condition can be detected before birth.*

INHERITING GENES

Half of a baby's genes come from his mother, via the ovum, and half come from his father, via the sperm.

Each ovum and sperm contains a different "mix" of the parents' genes, so each child inherits a unique selection of genetic information, which is different from that inherited by his siblings.

A gene can be dominant (it will always show up), or recessive, with 1 in 4 chances of showing up. So the dominant gene, say for brown eye colour, will prevail over a recessive, such as the gene for blue eyes.

The genetic mix
Your baby will be a unique combination of both parents' genes.

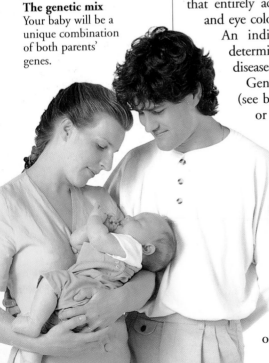

WHAT IS A GENE?

A gene is a minute unit of DNA (deoxyribonucleic acid) carried on a chromosome, which also consists of DNA. In the nucleus of every cell of the body, there are about 50,000 unique genes divided among 23 pairs of chromosomes.

THE "BLUEPRINT" OF THE BODY

Genes influence and direct the development and functioning of all the organs and body systems. They determine the pattern for growth, survival, reproduction and possibly ageing and death for each individual. Because all cells (except for the egg and sperm cells) derive from the single fertilized egg, the same genetic material is duplicated in every cell in your body. However, not all the genes contained within a cell are active; it is the site and function of the cell that determines which genes are active. For example, different sets of genes are active in bone and blood cells.

Except for identical twins, individuals differ greatly in the composition of their genes, and it is their genes that entirely account for any variation in height, hair and eye colour, body shape and gender, for example.

An individual's genetic inheritance will also determine his or her susceptibility to certain diseases and disorders.

Genes are held in pairs along a chromosome (see below) and each gene is either dominant or recessive. A recognizable effect is the result of the dominant gene or genes in each individual pair; the effect of recessive genes will only be noticeable when there are two recessive genes (see column, left).

Chromosomes Twenty-three pairs of these thread-like structures are present in the nucleus of every cell, except for the egg and sperm cells. These cells usually contain only 22 chromosomes plus an X or Y chromosome. Each chromosome contains thousands of genes arranged in single file along its length. Chromosomes are made up of two chains of DNA, which are arranged together to form a ladder-like structure. This spirals around upon itself and is known as a double helix (see below). DNA has four bases, which are arranged in varying combinations, each of which provides coded instructions to regulate all the activities of the body.

Chromosomal disorders are usually due to a fault in the process of chromosome division in the formation of the egg or sperm, or during the initial divisions of the fertilized ovum. Abnormalities of the sex chromosomes result in defects in sexual development, and cause infertility and occasionally mental retardation. Abnormalities can be diagnosed by chromosome analysis, one of the techniques used in genetic counselling (see p. 16).

MUTANT GENES

Sometimes when a cell divides and duplicates its genetic material, the copying process is not perfect, and a fault occurs. This leads to a small change, or mutation, in the structure of the genetic material.

Carrying a mutant gene normally has a neutral or harmless effect – most, if not all of us have a mutant gene as part of our genetic make-up. Occasionally, however, it can have a disadvantageous or, more rarely, a beneficial effect.

The effects of a mutant gene depend largely upon whether it is carried within the fused ovum and the sperm, or whether it is a fault in the later copying process of the cells (somatic or body cells).

A mutation in the ovum or sperm will reproduce itself in all of the body's cells, resulting in genetic diseases such as cystic fibrosis. A mutated somatic cell, at worst, will multiply to form a group of abnormal cells in a specific area. These may have only a minor local effect, or they may cause deformity or disease. This type of mutation is usually triggered by outside influences, such as radiation or exposure to carcinogens.

The double helix
The two chains of DNA, which make up each of the 46 chromosomes, are arranged to make a long spiralling ladder.

— Chromosome

Each of the four DNA bases – adenine, cytosine, guanine and thymine – is represented by a different colour

Sugar-phosphate molecules form the sides of the DNA ladder

Gene

DNA replication
When a new cell is about to be formed, the DNA in each of the chromosomes "unzips" along the centre of the ladder, and each half of DNA duplicates itself. The new chains created should be genetically identical to the original ones.

It is important to seek expert advice if you fall into any of the following groups:

• *If a previous child was born with a genetic disorder such as cystic fibrosis or haemophilia, or a chromosomal disorder such as Down's syndrome.*

• *If a previous child was born with a congenital defect, for example, a club foot.*

• *If there is a family history of mental disability, or abnormal physical development.*

• *If there is a blood relationship between you and your partner.*

• *If you have a history of repeated miscarriages.*

• *If either parent is over 35.*

GENETIC COUNSELLING

Genetic counselling is aimed at determining the risk you run of passing on an inheritable disease to your child or of having a child with a chromosomal defect because of your age. It also helps you to decide whether or not to go ahead and conceive in the light of that assessment. You may be particularly concerned because you have a blood relative (even, perhaps, a previous child) who has suffered from an inheritable disorder.

HOW GENETIC COUNSELLING WORKS

When you are referred for genetic counselling, the counsellor will ask both of you for details of your age, health and family backgrounds. Virtually every case is unique. The advice depends on a precise diagnosis of a known disease (what it is and why it occurred), and on the creation of a comprehensive family tree that details all blood relationships and any diseases suffered. Genetic counsellors are also trained in psychology: they will assess the degree of risk involved and help you make an informed decision. If the risk is small, you may decide to go ahead and try for a baby. If, however, the risk is high, you may prefer not to take a chance.

For many genetic disorders, such as sickle-cell anaemia or Tay-Sach's disease (see p. 13), it is possible to establish whether parents are carriers. This can be done by seeing the disease itself, such as sickle-shaped cells on a blood test; by looking for the product of the disease, such as the proteins that are present in Tay-Sach's; or by flagging a gene or chromosome. Flagging is a sophisticated technique that finds out if a fragment of DNA will attach itself to a chromosome. If it does, the gene, and therefore the disease, is present in your or your partner's genetic blueprint; if not, it is absent. However, in most diseases, more than one gene is involved, so it can be difficult to check all the elements. This is true of cystic fibrosis, for example, although at present the diagnosis can be over 90 percent certain.

If you already have an affected child, it is important to rule out a cause that is not inherited, such as rubella (see p. 11), exposure to radiation, drugs or injury. Sometimes it can be difficult to pinpoint the exact cause, but your chances of having another affected child will be outlined.

YOU ARE PREGNANT

As soon as you suspect that you might be pregnant you should seek confirmation. There is a variety of tests available that can be performed at different intervals after conception. Some are more accurate than others.

Blood test This test has to be performed by your doctor and is becoming more widely available. It can accurately detect the pregnancy hormone hCG (human chorionic gonadotrophin) in the blood as early as two weeks after conception – about the time your next period is due.

Urine tests HCG can also be detected in your urine. A urine test can be carried out by you at home, or by the hospital, your doctor's surgery, a family planning clinic or a pharmacy. They are over 90 percent reliable and can be performed as soon as two weeks after conception, although you will get the most reliable result if you wait four weeks longer.

ANTENATAL CARE

Consultations, check-ups and tests will be carried out throughout your pregnancy to monitor your health and that of your baby. Although most pregnancies proceed normally, these visits and investigations are vital to monitor progress and spot any potential problems early on.

The antenatal clinic You will attend the antenatal clinic either at the hospital where you plan to have your baby or at your doctor's surgery. Most women attend once a month up until week 28, every two weeks up to 36 weeks, and then once a week for the last month. If there are any complications, such as you are expecting more than one baby or you have a pre-existing medical condition, or if you are thought to be at risk, you will need to attend more frequently.

Attending an antenatal clinic in a large hospital can often seem intimidating and frustrating, especially if you see different nurses and doctors at every visit. This can be avoided if you opt for a GP clinic, or care by a community midwife, or shared care so that you mainly see your doctor or your midwife for check-ups with occasional visits to the hospital clinic for tests.

YOUR FILE

At your first antenatal visit you will be given a personal file or booklet. On it, details of your personal history (see below), the routine tests and progress of your pregnancy will be recorded by your doctor and midwives, as well as any special tests that you may have. This file goes with you at all times and you must remember to have it with you when you go into labour.

At the first visit you will be asked various questions on the following subjects:

- *Your personal details and circumstances.*
- *Childhood illnesses or serious illnesses you have had.*
- *Illnesses that run in your family, and also in your partner's family.*
- *If there are twins in your family.*
- *Your menstrual history – when you started, how long your average cycle is, how many days you bleed, and the date of your last period.*
- *What symptoms of pregnancy you have, and your general health.*
- *Details of any previous births, pregnancies, miscarriages or problems in conceiving.*
- *If you are taking any prescription medicine or if you suffer from any allergies.*

URINE AND BLOOD TESTS

At each visit your urine is tested and at your first visit a sample of blood is taken for various tests.

Urine tests *You will be asked to provide a sample of midstream urine. To do this, first clean the vulva with a sterile pad, and then pass the first few drops into the toilet bowl and collect a sample of the midstream urine in a sterile container.*

This is tested for signs of kidney infection and also for protein, which is a sign of urinary tract infection; for sugar, to check that you are not developing diabetes; and for ketones, which are the classic sign that diabetes is established and needs urgent treatment. A rare cause is very severe vomiting in pregnancy, called hyperemesis gravidarum, which requires urgent hospitalization.

Blood tests *At your first visit, a blood sample will be taken to find out the following:*

- *Your basic blood group (A, B, O, AB), and your Rhesus (Rh) blood group (positive or negative). If you are Rh negative, you will be tested for Rhesus incompatibility.*

- *Your haemoglobin level. This is a measure of the oxygen-carrying power of your red blood cells.*

- *To check for rubella (German measles) – to see whether or not you are immune to this disease.*

ROUTINE ANTENATAL CHECKS

Every pregnant woman has certain routine checks to establish her state of health and the condition of her baby. They may be performed at every visit, or at different times during her pregnancy. Some are performed only once. If the tests indicate there is, or that there may be, a problem, you will be monitored closely and prompt action will be taken if necessary.

Height and shoe size Your height will be measured at your first visit and your shoe size may be noted. If you are very petite with small feet, you may also have a small pelvic inlet and outlet, both of which need to be assessed. However, it is likely that your baby will be exactly right for your particular physical build.

Weight Your weight is noted at most visits. In the first trimester a loss of weight usually reflects nausea and vomiting due to morning sickness and is usually nothing to worry about. Sudden weight gain may reflect fluid retention and indicate pre-eclampsia. In the past, maternal weight gain was taken as a reliable indicator of the growth of the baby. Research now indicates, however, that maternal weight gain alone should not be relied upon, but viewed in conjunction with external and internal examinations, blood and urinary tests and ultrasound scans.

Breasts Your breasts are examined, and the condition of your nipples is noted. A very few women have dimpled, or inverted nipples and these can be corrected by wearing a breastshield inside your bra, although they usually correct themselves during pregnancy.

External examination At every visit your abdomen is gently felt and measured to determine the size of the baby. This assessment gives a good idea of whether your baby is the right size for your dates, and an accurate picture of your baby's rate of development. The top (fundus) of your uterus is routinely felt, and after 12 weeks the distance between your pelvic bone and the top of your uterus is measured. The amount of amniotic fluid, as well as your individual size and weight, can affect the reading, so after 26 weeks, the baby's "poles" (head and rump) are also felt.

CHILDBIRTH CLASSES

As an enthusiastic proponent of prepared childbirth, I believe that everyone can benefit from childbirth classes. These classes can be tremendously enjoyable. The camaraderie is wonderful, and you may find the other members of the group act as a substitute for your extended family as you exchange folklore; certainly they will make you feel less alone and isolated. It's a great help to be able to share feelings and experiences with people who are in the same position and it can help relieve tension and anxiety. Strong personal bonds are often formed with others in the class that can be the basis of lasting friendships for you and your baby.

PREPARATION FOR PARENTING

Classes that teach childbirth and parentcraft are particularly useful for first-time parents because they're designed to give you information that will make you both feel more confident not only during labour and birth but also when you have your new baby to care for. They work in three ways:

First, they cover the processes of pregnancy and birth, including female anatomy and physiology, and the changes that occur throughout pregnancy. This is so that you will have a clearer understanding of what is involved and why certain changes are taking place. The teacher will talk you through the stages of labour, the birth and your postnatal recovery and explain what medical procedures you can expect, and why these are carried out.

Second, they provide instruction in relaxation, breathing and exercise techniques that will help you control your labour, reduce pain, and give you the confidence that only comes when you are familiar with what is going to happen. Bear in mind that bodies, not brains, give birth, so anything that helps you tune into your body is going to be useful. Your partner also learns about being a supportive birth attendant (see column, p. 20) and how to give you a massage to help relieve your pain (see p. 40).

Finally, you will be advised on breastfeeding and offered practice in the practicalities of caring for your newborn; this will include bathing and dressing the baby, changing nappies, making up formula and bottlefeeding.

CHOOSING CHILDBIRTH CLASSES

Both the quality and approach of childbirth classes can vary – some are tightly structured with little question-and-answer time, others allow time to practise techniques. Some depend mainly on lectures, others on class participation.

The teacher is usually the determining factor, so talk to the teacher and, if you can, check with other couples who have attended a particular class before you make your final choice. Try to select a teacher whose philosophy of birth fits in with the type of birth you'd like to have, or conflicts and confusion can arise later during labour.

Find out how many couples are taught in each class. Half a dozen couples is an ideal size since you will receive plenty of attention from the teacher while being intimate with your fellow participants.

You will have to consider antenatal classes fairly early in your pregnancy because in some cases you need to book a place; make plans to start the classes in your eighth month.

Strengthening the muscles used in childbirth often results in an easier delivery. Many hospitals and independent organizations offer classes that also incorporate exercise and relaxation classes – some will prepare you for specific types of birth.

19

FATHER'S ROLE

In an antenatal class you may be able to show your partner for the first time just how important a role he is going to have.

By familiarizing him with the processes of labour and delivery, childbirth classes will give your partner the chance to be an effective birth assistant.

Some courses also provide father-only sessions where the men can talk freely about any problems or anxieties they have about the forthcoming event. A nervous partner should also find security and support in the company of other fathers-to-be.

Team effort *Childbirth classes give a couple a unique opportunity to work as a team towards a common goal – the birth of their baby – and very often this results in a special closeness.*

Partners can help
At classes, your partner can learn how to massage your back during the early stages of labour.

TECHNIQUES OF CHILDBIRTH CLASSES

Many studies have shown that taking childbirth classes shortens the length of labour. This is probably because knowing how to deal with pain produces a more relaxed labour. Strategies taught at childbirth classes that deal with labour pain include the following:

Cognitive control This works by disassociating your mind from the pain you are experiencing. You visualize a pleasant scenario in which you feel happy about experiencing contractions; for example, when you feel pain you imagine your baby moving further down the birth canal, closer to emerging. In this way, you concentrate on the positive element of the sensation.

You can also use distraction to cope with pain, although this works best in the early stages. To take your mind off the pain, and prevent it from completely filling your consciousness and overwhelming you, try counting to twenty, going through a list of possible names for your new baby, or concentrating on a beautiful picture or piece of music. Focusing your attention on breathing techniques and becoming aware of your breathing pattern is another way of forcing your mind away from the pain.

Systematic relaxation In order to decrease your fear of pain and thus increase your tolerance of it, you are taught exercises to relax the various muscles of the body. In this way you are able to isolate the pain of contractions rather than allowing it to pervade the whole of your body.

Hawthorne rehearsal During your labour you receive enhanced attention from a birth assistant. Psychological research has shown that the more attention you are given, the less pain you feel.

Systematic desensitization You gradually become more tolerant of pain. This technique involves your partner pinching your leg very hard at every antenatal class to illustrate how painful a contraction can be so that by the end of the course you can tolerate pain for longer periods.

CHAPTER 2

DIET IN PREGNANCY

Your body will never work harder than it does during pregnancy and childbirth. To cope with the increased physical needs, maintain your strength and energy levels, and give your baby the best start in life, you must eat well. Eating healthily is mainly a question of having a wide variety of the right kind of foods – those rich in essential nutrients – and avoiding high-calorie foods that contain mostly sugar, refined carbohydrates or fats. Make sure your diet includes lots of fresh fruit and vegetables, whole grains, protein and low-fat dairy produce to maintain your own and your baby's good health.

EATING FOR YOURSELF

During pregnancy and childbirth your body will have to work much harder than it does normally. To cope with the extra demands, maintain your strength and enjoy your pregnancy, you must eat well.

• *Increase your intake by 500 calories per day.*

• *Start to eat 5–6 small meals a day instead of 2–3 big ones.*

• *Make certain you eat extra protein and carbohydrates (see p. 26); protein supplies essential nutrients for your developing baby, carbohydrates meet your energy needs.*

• *Eat foods that are rich in vitamins and minerals, especially iron (see p. 27) – essential for healthy organs.*

Gaining weight
Doctors recommend that a woman of average weight, experiencing an average pregnancy, ought to gain approximately 10–14kg (20–28lb) in the total 40 weeks gestation as shown in the chart (right). This allows about 3–4kg (6–8lb) for the baby and about 7–10kg (14–20lb) for the baby's support system (placenta, amniotic fluid, increased blood, fluid, fat and breast tissue). It is usual to gain very little, if anything, during the first trimester, approximately 0.5–1kg (1–2lb) each week in months 4–8, then very little in the last month.

FOOD IN PREGNANCY

Pregnant women, like most people, rarely have the time or inclination to begin measuring out ounces of this and portions of that and trying to remember the calorific value of everything. In fact, there's no need to do this as long as you follow some basic guidelines given in the following pages about healthy eating in pregnancy. In many ways, good nutrition is just common sense.

EATING FOR TWO?

As your pregnancy progresses your appetite will increase; this is nature's way of making certain you eat enough for you and your baby. Your energy requirements will increase only by 25 percent, or 500 calories per day, far less than if you ate twice your normal amount of food. (Certain mothers-to-be, however, such as those who previously ate an inadequate or unbalanced diet, may have special requirements.) The saying "eating for two", therefore, merely underlines your responsibility to provide for the nutritional needs of your developing baby. Pregnancy is not the time for dieting. Research has shown that when mothers-to-be eat poor diets, there is a higher incidence of serious problems than normal.

AVERAGE WEIGHT GAIN IN PREGNANCY

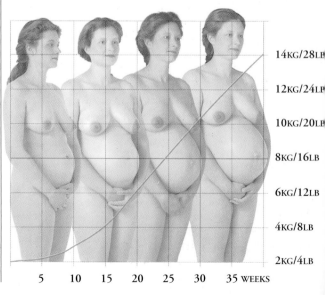

14KG/28LB
12KG/24LB
10KG/20LB
8KG/16LB
6KG/12LB
4KG/8LB
2KG/4LB

5   10   15   20   25   30   35 WEEKS

However, you do need to beware of really excess weight gain; fat that is deposited at the tops of the arms and the thighs is very difficult to get rid of after pregnancy. A quite substantial amount of fat will be lost by breastfeeding your baby, as it is accumulated specifically to be converted to milk during lactation. However, some will remain and this will be difficult to lose once you have finished breastfeeding.

You therefore owe it to yourself, as well as your baby, to eat a diet that is best for both of you. While you should adhere to the nutritional recommendations on pages 28 and 29, you can balance your food intake over a 24- to 48-hour period rather than at each meal.

BABY'S REQUIREMENTS

During pregnancy, you are your baby's only source of nourishment. Every calorie, vitamin, or gram of protein that your baby needs must be eaten by you. You will fulfil all of your baby's requirements when you eat red meat (if you eat it), fresh fruit, vegetables, eggs, beans, peas, wholemeal pasta and cereals, fish, fowl and low-fat dairy products. (A Danish study has shown that eating oil-rich fish – salmon, herring, sardine – may help lessen the risk of preterm birth.) Make your diet as varied as possible, choosing from a wide range of foods.

WHAT YOU NEED

You are the other important person you must eat for during pregnancy. A good diet will mean that you have better reserves to cope with, and recover from, the indisputable strain of pregnancy and the hard work of labour. Anaemia and pre-eclampsia are much more common in those mothers who have a poor diet, and some problems, such as morning sickness and leg cramps, may be exacerbated by what you do or don't eat – not eating enough calcium, for example, is thought to cause leg cramps.

Overall, good nutrition will help minimize excessive mood swings, constipation, fatigue and other common complaints (see pp. 62–70). In addition, a sensible eating regime that cuts out or restricts the amount of empty calories that you consume will mean that you will put on less weight and be left with less excess fat to lose after your child has been born.

EMPTY CALORIES

The following foods should be reduced in pregnancy; they usually contain nothing more than sugar or sugar substitutes and refined flour.

- *Any form of sweetener – including white or brown sugar, golden syrup, treacle and artificial products such as saccharine and aspartame.*

- *Sweets and chocolate bars.*

- *Soft drinks, such as cola and sweetened fruit juices.*

- *Commercially produced biscuits, cakes, pastries, doughnuts and pies, as well as jam and marmalade.*

- *Tinned fruit in syrup.*

- *Artificial cream.*

- *Sweetened breakfast cereal.*

- *Ice cream and sorbets that contain added sugar. Freeze fruit juice or puréed fruit instead.*

- *Savouries that contain sugar, such as peanut butter, relishes, pickles, salad dressings, mayonnaise, spaghetti sauces and many others – read the label to check the sugar content.*

YOUR OFFICE SUPPLIES

The average nine-to-five job can wreak havoc with your nutritional intake. However, forward planning and a few strategically situated supplies can help.

In the office refrigerator
- *Mineral water.*
- *Unsweetened fruit juice.*
- *Plain live-culture yogurt.*
- *Dutch or Swiss cheese.*
- *Hard-boiled eggs.*
- *Fresh fruit.*
- *Vegetable snacks – carrot and red pepper sticks, tomatoes.*
- *Wholemeal bread.*
- *Jar of wheatgerm.*

In your desk drawer
- *Wholemeal crackers, crispbreads, or breadsticks, perhaps with seeds.*
- *Dried fruit.*
- *Nuts or seeds.*
- *Decaffeinated instant coffee and decaffeinated tea bags.*
- *Powdered skimmed milk for extra calcium in drinks.*

In your handbag
- *Wholemeal crackers, crispbreads or breadsticks, perhaps with seeds.*
- *Dried fruit, nuts and seeds.*
- *Fresh fruit or vegetable snacks.*
- *Small thermos of unsweetened juice or milk.*

WHAT TO EAT

Quality food is as close to its original state as possible and offers you and your baby good nutritional value. Your goal should be to eat quality food throughout your pregnancy and afterwards, especially if you breastfeed.

When shopping, select fresh produce; seasonal fruit and vegetables will be fresher as well as cheaper. Always wash fruit and vegetables thoroughly before use. To avoid the risk of contracting a food-related illness, do not eat liver, unpasteurized cheeses and cook-chill dishes, particularly if they contain seafood and pork (see p. 30). If you can afford it, opt for free-range or organic foods that are free from pesticides and hormones.

Frozen packets of vegetables, such as peas and runner beans, are good stand-bys – particularly when vegetables are out of season – but avoid canned food, except for plum tomatoes and oily fish.

Foods that have been over-refined, such as white flour and white sugar, have had all of the natural goodness stripped out of them and can offer you and your baby nothing but excess calories. Instead, choose wholemeal bread, pastry and flour, rather than "enriched" refined products, as it is highly unlikely that the enrichment puts back in all that has been taken out. The two "waste" products of refining are bran (the fibre) and wheatgerm (the heart of the wheat) and these contain most of the goodness. The addition of bran may help prevent constipation (as long as you don't mind the taste) and everyone can benefit from the multitude of vitamins and minerals in wheatgerm. Wheatgerm tastes a bit like bean sprouts – crunchy and nutty – and can be added to all kinds of dishes. It is available from healthfood shops, and should be kept in the refrigerator after opening.

As you'll probably have good days with energy and low days when you won't want to bother, cook up a large batch of meals when you are feeling energetic, and store them in the freezer or pantry, to be used when you're too tired to cook. Banish junk food from your kitchen.

IF YOU ARE A VEGETARIAN

A number of people do not eat animal products; many more people who aren't strict vegetarians limit their intake of meat, particularly red meat. If you fall into one of these categories, you need to make special efforts to ensure you eat enough protein, vitamins and iron to meet your own and your baby's needs (see also p. 28).

Non-meat eaters can get their protein from eggs, cheese, milk and fish, but if you do not eat these you will need to make up for this by eating incomplete but complementary plant protein sources such as pulses and whole grains. These, when eaten in combination, will provide you with most of the necessary amino acids normally found complete in animal forms of protein (see below). For extra calcium, all pregnant women should increase their intake of milk to half a litre (a pint) a day (choose semi-skimmed milk which has all the calcium but less fat than whole milk).

All vegetarians need to make sure they take in sufficient iron because there is relatively little in vegetables, and certain substances interfere with its absorption (see p. 26). Eggs and green leafy vegetables will provide iron, but not as much as you get from red meat.

If you eat no animal products at all, you will have to work harder to make sure that you are not deficient in calcium, vitamins B^6, B^{12} and D, all of which are provided by meat and dairy products. Vitamin B^{12} is only found in animal sources; although very little is needed, lack of it will eventually lead to pernicious anaemia. If your diet contains no animal protein, it is essential that you take vitamin B^{12} supplements.

SHORT CUTS

When time, energy or money are short, eating nutritiously can often seem to be too much hassle. Here are some tips that will help you do the best for you and your baby, without too much effort.

- *Keep a supply of various frozen vegetables.*

- *Buy meat and fish in bulk, and freeze in meal-size portions.*

- *Cook ahead and freeze.*

- *Buy ready-made fresh salads.*

- *A microwave oven cooks food quickly and retains nutrients.*

- *Keep it simple – eat raw vegetables and fruit; steam, stir fry or grill for speed, or bake so you can leave food to cook on its own.*

- *Enlist help – many grandparents-to-be will undoubtedly be itching to lend you a hand.*

COMPLEMENTARY PROTEINS

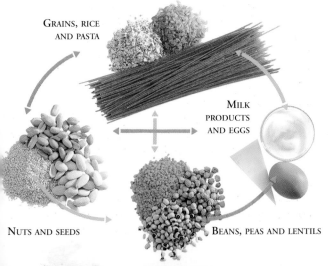

GRAINS, RICE AND PASTA

MILK PRODUCTS AND EGGS

NUTS AND SEEDS

BEANS, PEAS AND LENTILS

Combining proteins

All animal products contribute complete proteins, so called because they contain all the essential amino acids that the body needs in the right proportions. Plant products contribute incomplete proteins, and to get the full complement of necessary amino acids, you have to eat certain foods in combination. For example, peas with rice or pasta; a handful of nuts with rice and beans.

◄▷ GENERALLY COMPLEMENTARY

◄▮▷ SOMETIMES COMPLEMENTARY

25

CHOOSING PROTEINS

Due to the intensive development of your baby, your protein requirement increases by over 65 percent from the onset of pregnancy.

This means your needs jump from 45–60g (1½–2¼oz) to 75–100g (2⅔–3½oz) of protein daily, depending on how active you are.

Proteins are made up of amino acids, which are vital to individual body cells and tissues. A total of 20 different amino acids are required. The body can synthesize 12 of these, the non-essential amino acids, but eight others, the essential acids, must be supplied by the food you eat. These latter are found only in complete proteins in animal products such as meat, dairy products, fish, poultry and eggs. Always choose organically reared produce, especially poultry, eggs and beef whenever possible.

You also need to be guided by what else you are getting from protein-rich food. Meat is the richest source of complete proteins and also contains vital B vitamins. However, some meat, particularly red meat, can be very high in animal fat, so you could choose fish instead. Fish has complete proteins and is high in vitamins and nutritious fish oils, and low in fat.

Equivalent amounts of protein are one egg, one slice of hard cheese, 2 tablespoons peanut butter, 2 tablespoons cottage cheese, ½ cup peas or beans.

ESSENTIAL NUTRITION

Research has found that what you eat when you are pregnant not only affects your baby at birth, but also appears to have a long-term effect throughout your child's life – even into old age.

PROTEIN

Protein is probably the most essential nutrient for your baby; the amino acids that make up protein are literally the building blocks of the body. Proteins form the main structural elements of the cells and tissues that make up muscles, bones, connective tissues and also many of your vital organs such as the heart, lungs and kidneys.

The type and quality of protein in food varies (see column, left). Generally, the more expensive foodstuffs like meat, fish and poultry are the best sources, but cheaper products eaten together can also supply you with adequate protein. Wholewheat bread or pasta with beans, cheese, eggs or peanut butter; or brown rice or noodles with sesame seeds, nuts, and milk are cheaper ingredients that will provide your protein intake. You need at least three servings of protein (see p. 28) daily.

CARBOHYDRATES AND CALORIES

These should provide the largest part of your daily calorie intake. As you need to increase your calorie intake by 500 calories a day during pregnancy, you should make certain that you eat the best (unrefined) carbohydrates that you can and avoid empty calories.

Simple carbohydrates are sugars in various forms. The most common types and sources are sucrose (cane sugar), glucose (honey), fructose (fruit), and maltose, lactose and galactose (milk sugars). Because they are absorbed quickly from the stomach, all provide "instant energy". This is useful when you are in dire need (glucose sweets may also be helpful if you have nausea).

Complex carbohydrates are the starches contained in grains, potatoes, lentils, beans and peas. The body has to break them down into simple carbohydrates before it can use them, so they provide a steady supply of energy over a longer period of time. In addition, complex unrefined carbohydrates (such as wholemeal oats and brown rice) provide fibre, vitamins and minerals.

VITAMINS

These are essential for health. Good sources of many vitamins (and minerals) are vegetables and fruits. Some are rich in vitamin C and others contain vitamins A, B, E and folic acid; you must include them all in your daily diet. Many vitamins are fragile, and are quickly destroyed by exposure to light, air and heat. Some cannot be stored in the body, so good quantities must be eaten every day. Leafy green and yellow/red vegetables and fruit supply vitamins A, E, B^6, (as well as minerals iron, zinc and magnesium).

Although some B vitamins are supplied by vegetables and fruit, the bulk of our vitamin B intake is usually supplied by meat, fish, dairy products, grains and nuts. Some are entirely from animal products, so vegetarians must take extra care to make sure they fulfil their nutritional requirements (see p. 24).

MINERALS

Minerals and trace elements are essential for the proper functioning of the body but cannot be synthesized by it. A varied diet should supply you with sufficient amounts. Two in particular, iron and calcium, must be consumed at high levels to support your baby's development.

Iron Essential for the production of haemoglobin (the oxygen-carrying part of the red blood cells) its intake must not only be adequate (see column, right) but continuous during pregnancy. Bear in mind that iron, particularly iron supplements, can block the absorption of zinc, which is also essential for the development of your baby's brain and nervous system. So you should eat zinc-rich foods, such as fish and wheatgerm, separately from iron-rich foods.

Calcium Your baby's bones begin to form between weeks four and six, so it's absolutely crucial that your intake of calcium is high prior to pregnancy, and remains high throughout the rest of pregnancy. Foods rich in calcium include all dairy products (choose low-fat ones), powdered milk, green leafy vegetables, soya products, broccoli, and any bony fish such as sardines and whitebait. If you can't drink milk or eat dairy products, you may need supplements.

GETTING ENOUGH IRON

Necessary iron intake varies from woman to woman and the form in which it is best taken is open to debate.

The preferred way of ingesting iron is from foods such as eggs and organically-reared red meat. These animal sources of iron are more easily absorbed than iron from fruit and vegetables. It is advisable to avoid liver during pregnancy because liver contains high levels of vitamin A that may be toxic to the fetus.

Iron-rich foods, besides the above, include fish, haricot beans, apricots, raisins and prunes.

If you are iron-deficient when you become pregnant, or develop iron deficiency later on, iron tablets or injections will be prescribed by your doctor to prevent anaemia.

VITAMIN D

This is required to help calcium absorption, so some of your daily intake should come from cheese and eggs – food in which both are present. Vitamin D can be produced by the body if it is triggered by the action of sunlight on the skin.

• *Most pale-skinned people need about 40 minutes of sunlight a day.*

• *Dark-skinned people who live far from the equator, need progressively more depending on their skin tones.*

YOUR DAILY NEEDS

Although there is no need for you to become obsessive about calculating your daily food intake, it is good to have a guide to be sure that you are eating and drinking as well as you possibly can. If you prefer, you can work out your nutritional intake over the course of two days, rather than balancing each meal.

YOUR FLUID INTAKE

During pregnancy your blood volume and blood fluids will expand by nearly half, so it is very important to keep up your fluid intake. Do not restrict it at all except for cutting out high-calorie drinks. Water is best, although fruit juices are good, too. If you suffer from mild swelling of the ankles, face or fingers, it will not help to limit your fluid intake. However, it is also essential to keep up your salt intake to avoid problems of salt depletion.

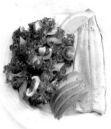

Healthy eating
When you do not feel like eating large meals, you can eat lightly but well if you stick to fish, salads and fruit. Milk provides necessary calcium.

A HEALTHY DIET

FOOD TYPES	SUGGESTED SOURCES	
Calcium foods	200ml/⅓ pint milk or milk made up from powdered milk 75g/3oz tinned sardines, with bones	50g/2oz hard cheese 100g/4oz soft cheese 325g/13oz cottage cheese 255ml/9fl oz yoghurt
First-class protein foods	100g/4oz fresh or tinned fish 100g/4oz prawns 75g/3oz beef, lamb, pork, poultry or offal (not liver), without the fat	75g/3oz hard cheese 100g/4oz soft cheese 600ml/1 pint milk 340ml/12fl oz yoghurt 3 eggs, size 1
Green leafy and yellow/red vegetables and fruits for vitamins and minerals	50g/2oz melon 6 plums 1 mango, orange or grapefruit 2 apricots 4 peaches, apples or pears	25g/1oz spinach or broccoli 13g/½oz carrots 250g/10oz peas or beans 25g/1oz sweet peppers 150g/6oz tomatoes
Whole grains and complex carbohydrates	75g/3oz kidney beans, soya beans or chick peas 100g/4oz lentils or peas 1 wholemeal pitta or tortilla 6 wholemeal biscuits	75g/3oz cooked barley, brown rice, millet or bulgar wheat 25g/1oz wholemeal or soya flour 1 slice wholemeal or soya bread 6 wholemeal bread sticks
Vitamin C foods	25g/1oz blackcurrants 75g/3oz strawberries 1 large lemon or orange ½ medium grapefruit	25g/1oz sweet peppers 225g/9oz tomatoes 200g/8oz blackberries or raspberries 115ml/4fl oz citrus juice

VITAMIN AND MINERAL SOURCES

We are dependent on food sources for all our vitamin and mineral needs, except for vitamin D. The chart below is a guide to the best sources of essential vitamins and minerals. These tend to be fragile, so always try to eat foods that are as fresh as possible.

SOURCES OF VITAMINS AND MINERALS

NAME	FOOD SOURCE
Vitamin A	Milk, butter, cheese, egg yolks, oily fish, offal (avoid liver), green/yellow fruit and vegetables
Vitamin B^1	Whole grains, nuts, pulses, offal (avoid liver), pork, brewer's yeast, wheatgerm
Vitamin B^2	Brewer's yeast, wheatgerm, whole grains, green vegetables, milk, cheese, eggs
Vitamin B^3	Brewer's yeast, whole grains, wheatgerm, offal (avoid liver), green vegetables, oily fish, eggs
Vitamin B^5	Kidneys, eggs, peanuts, whole grains, cheese
Vitamin B^6	Brewer's yeast, whole grains, soya flour, wheatgerm, mushrooms, potatoes, avocados
Vitamin B^{12}	Meat, offal (not liver), fish, milk, eggs
Folic acid	Raw leafy vegetables, peas, soya flour, oranges, bananas, walnuts
Vitamin C	Rosehip syrup, sweet peppers, citrus fruits, blackcurrants, tomatoes
Vitamin D	Fortified milk, oily fish, eggs (particularly the yolks), butter
Vitamin E	Wheatgerm, egg yolks, peanuts, seeds, vegetable oils, broccoli
Calcium	Milk, cheese, small fish with bones, peanuts, walnuts, sunflower seeds, yoghurt, broccoli
Iron	Kidneys, fish, egg yolks, red meat, cereals, molasses, apricots, haricot beans
Zinc	Wheatbran, eggs, nuts, onions, shellfish, sunflower seeds, wheatgerm, whole grains

YOUR DAILY REQUIREMENTS

To give you and your baby the best possible diet, try to include as many of the following foods every day, choosing from the chart of suggested sources (opposite). Each of the suggested sources represents a single serving. Try to vary the types of food that you eat.

- *First-class proteins (meat, poultry, fish, eggs, cheese and dairy products) – 3 servings.*

- *Green leafy and yellow/red vegetables and fruits – 3 servings.*

- *Other fruit and vegetables – 1 or 2 servings.*

- *Calcium foods (dairy products, fish with bones) – 4 servings in pregnancy, 5 during breastfeeding.*

- *Whole grains and complex carbohydrates (wholemeal bread and biscuits, whole grain rice and pasta, beans and pulses) – 4 or 5 servings.*

- *Iron-rich food (red meat, egg yolks, apricots and haricot beans) – 2 servings.*

- *Fluids – 8 glasses a day, preferably not coffee or alcohol. Water is best.*

FOOD SAFETY

Scrupulous kitchen hygiene is essential because some illnesses are dangerous during pregnancy. Never take risks when handling and storing food; keep food cold at all times because bacteria can multiply rapidly in warm conditions.

• *Always use clean utensils between jobs or tastings.*

• *Always wash hands after going to the lavatory and before touching food, and take good care to cover any infections or cuts.*

• *Ensure that all frozen food, especially poultry and pork, is completely defrosted and thoroughly cooked.*

• *Never let raw meat or eggs come into contact with other foods. Wash your hands after touching these.*

• *Avoid dented and rusty tins.*

• *Avoid any food that looks or smells "off".*

• *Avoid soft cheeses and unpasteurized milk. If you do eat dairy products, make sure they are pasteurized.*

• *Do not refreeze food that has already been defrosted.*

• *Reheat food thoroughly only once, then throw away any leftover food.*

• *Do not eat liver or liver patés during pregnancy because they are high in vitamin A, which is known to be harmful when eaten in large quantities.*

FOODS TO AVOID

Food safety is important to help prevent illness and infections, so it makes sense to observe certain kitchen hygiene rules and avoid potentially harmful ingredients.

Processed foods Avoid foods containing chemicals – in particular, processed cheese and meats, cheese spreads and sausages. Do not eat highly salted foods, particularly those containing monosodium glutamate (MSG), which can cause dehydration and headaches.

Preserved food Avoid smoked fish, meat and cheese, pickled food and sausages. These often contain nitrate; an active agent that can react with the haemoglobin in your blood, thus reducing its oxygen-carrying power.

Drinks Caffeine is a stimulant and drinks containing it such as tea, coffee and chocolate should be avoided in pregnancy. The tannin in tea interferes with iron absorption, so avoid drinking too much.

FOOD HAZARDS

Certain precautions should be taken because we now know that some foods are contaminated with enough numbers of bacteria to cause illness, and may even cause miscarriage or birth defects.

Listeriosis Listeria is a rare bacterium found in soft cheeses, unpasteurized milk, ready-made coleslaw, cooked chilled foods, pâtés and improperly cooked meat. Bacteria are normally destroyed at pasteurizing temperatures, but if food is infected and refrigerated, the bacteria may continue to multiply. Also wash your hands after any direct contact with infected animals, such as sheep.

Salmonella This is a bacterium found in eggs and chicken that causes fever, abdominal pain and severe diarrhoea. It is killed by thorough cooking.

Toxoplasmosis This is caused by a parasite found in cat and dog faeces, and also in raw meat. It can cause birth defects. Always wash your hands after handling a pet or its litter tray, and wear gloves when gardening.

EXERCISE FOR PREGNANCY

Maintaining your physical and emotional energy levels during pregnancy is of prime importance. Exercising helps you stay in physical condition both before and after the birth. The benefits of exercise – improving your stamina, suppleness, strength and sense of well-being – will help you face the extra strain on your body as it adapts to meet the demands of pregnancy. It will also help counteract the tendency to feel clumsy or ungainly in the later months. With exercise, you can also develop a better understanding of your body's capabilities and learn different ways of relaxing, so that you can approach labour with confidence.

Exercising regularly can be emotionally as well as physically satisfying. It's an enjoyable way of preparing for the months of change ahead.

• *You will receive an emotional lift from the release of internal hormones such as endorphins.*

• *You will feel more contented, as the release of tranquillizing hormones that follows exercise aids relaxation.*

• *You can improve your self-awareness as you learn how to use your body in new ways.*

• *Backache, leg cramp, constipation and breathlessness can be alleviated by regular exercise.*

• *Your energy level will be increased.*

• *You will be better prepared for the work of labour.*

• *You will regain your shape more quickly after delivery.*

• *You can make new friends by meeting other mothers-to-be at antenatal exercise classes.*

• *You can share the exercise routine with your partner or other members of your family.*

GETTING FIT FOR PREGNANCY

The physical benefits of exercise – improving your stamina, suppleness and strength – will help you face the extra strain placed on your body as it adapts to meet the demands of pregnancy and childbirth. By exercising you can also develop a better understanding of your body's capabilities and learn different ways of relaxing.

Psychologically, exercising counteracts the tendency to feel clumsy, fat, or ungainly, particularly in the last three months. It increases your circulation, and that can help to ease tension. Labour may be easier and more comfortable if you have good muscle tone, and many of the exercises taught in antenatal classes, combined with relaxation and breathing techniques, will help you trust your body during labour. Staying in condition during pregnancy will also mean that you should regain your normal shape more quickly after your baby's birth.

HOW OFTEN

Incorporating a daily exercise routine into your busy schedule may not be very appealing. But many of the exercises recommended during pregnancy, as shown on the following pages, can usually be performed while you carry on with other activities: pelvic floor exercises may be performed while cleaning your teeth; foot and ankle exercises while sitting at your desk or on the bus; and tailor sitting while reading a book or watching television.

A little exercise several times a day is better than a lot of exercise all at once, and then none at all. Normally a woman can restore her energy by resting for half an hour, but it can take a pregnant woman half a day to recover from fatigue. So be kind to yourself and choose an activity that you will find enjoyable and relaxing.

WHAT YOU CAN DO

You are free to be involved in most sports during pregnancy (until the last trimester), as long as it is a sport you have been doing regularly beforehand, and you pursue it regularly once you are pregnant so that your body stays in condition. There are also activities that are particularly recommended during pregnancy (see opposite).

Walking Walking is good for the digestion, the circulation and your figure. Try to walk tall, with your buttocks tucked under, your shoulders back and keep your head up. Towards the end of pregnancy, however, you may find that the pelvic joint ligaments soften so much that you get backache if you walk more than a short distance. Always wear well-cushioned flat shoes.

Swimming This tones most muscles and is excellent for improving stamina. Because your weight is supported by the water, it is very difficult to strain muscles and joints, so swimming rarely results in physical injury. Some sports centres offer special antenatal work-out classes.

Yoga This has many benefits, such as increasing suppleness and reducing tension. It also teaches you to control your breathing and aids concentration during labour, which is very useful. Always tell the instructor that you are pregnant before taking any classes.

WHAT IS RISKY

Some sports, such as skiing and horseback riding, should not be attempted once you get big because your balance is thrown out by the new weight in front, and the chances of falling are high. Other activities, including those listed below, should be avoided because they put your body under unnecessary strain.

Jogging Don't jog while pregnant. It is very hard on your breasts (which need extra support during pregnancy) and jarring for your back, spine, pelvis, hips and knees.

Backpacking Weight-bearing activities are harmful because they put a severe strain on the ligaments in your back – and ligaments remain stretched, unlike muscles, which can return to their old shape.

Sit-ups Don't attempt these. The longitudinal muscles of the abdomen are designed to separate in the middle to allow room for the enlarging uterus, and sitting straight up from a lying position encourages them to part even further. The strain may slow down the recovery of abdominal tone after delivery. Leg lifts while you are lying on your back can have the same effect.

IS IT GOOD FOR YOUR BABY?

During exercise, your blood flow is optimum so every time you exercise within your limit, your baby gets a surge of oxygen into her blood. All her tissues, especially her brain, function in top form.

* *The hormones that are released during exercise pass across the placenta and reach your baby. At the beginning of exercise, therefore, your baby receives a lift from your adrenaline.*

* *During exercise, your baby also experiences the effect of endorphins, our own natural morphine-like substances that make us feel extremely good.*

* *The motion of exercise is extremely soothing, and your baby feels comforted from the rocking movements.*

EXERCISE WITH CARE

Begin your routine at a gentle pace, gradually building up to what feels right for you. Before each exercise, try a few deep breaths. This gets the blood flowing around your body and gives all your muscles a good supply of oxygen.

If you suffer any pain, cramping, or shortness of breath, stop exercising; when you resume, make sure it is at a slower pace. If you are out of breath, your baby is also being deprived of oxygen.

A gentle warm-up routine prepares your body for more demanding exercises and can easily be fitted into your daily life.

Warming up helps to relieve tension. It gently warms up muscles and joints and prevents your muscles becoming strained, thus reducing the risk of injury. You may suffer from cramp and later stiffness if you don't warm up.

STRETCHING

Before beginning any exercise routine always warm up gently (see column left) with these few stretching exercises. They will stimulate your blood circulation, giving you and your baby a good supply of oxygen. Repeat each exercise five to ten times; make sure you are comfortable and that your posture is good.

HEAD AND NECK EXERCISES

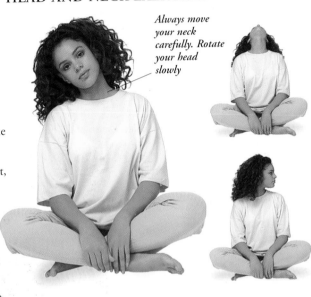

Always move your neck carefully. Rotate your head slowly

Head and neck
Gently tilt your head over to one side, then lift your chin and rotate your head gently over to the other side and down. Repeat, starting from the other side. Keeping your head straight, turn it slowly to the right, back to the front, and then to the left. Return to face the front.

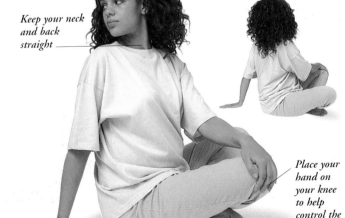

Keep your neck and back straight

Place your hand on your knee to help control the stretch

Waist
Sit comfortably with your legs crossed, straighten your back and gently stretch your neck upwards. Breathe out and turn your upper body to the right, placing your right hand behind you. Place your left hand on your right knee and use this hand as a lever to twist your body a little further, gently stretching the muscles of your waist. Repeat in the other direction.

STRETCHING YOUR SHOULDERS AND LEGS

Clasp your hands together lightly if you can; if you can't reach, don't worry

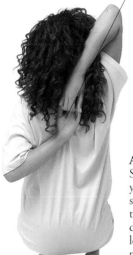

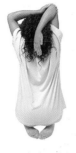

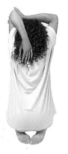

Arms and shoulders

Sit with your legs tucked under, lift your right arm up and slowly stretch it to the ceiling. Bend it at the elbow and drop your hand down behind your back. Put your left hand on your right elbow, pushing it further down. Put your left arm down behind your back and reach up to grasp the right hand. Stretch for 20 seconds, then relax. Repeat with other arm.

Legs and feet

Sit with your back straight and your legs stretched out in front of you. Place your hands on the floor next to your hips to support your weight. Bend your knee slowly and then straighten. Repeat with other leg. This will tone the muscles in your calf and thigh.

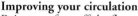

Keep your back straight and your weight central

Improving your circulation

Raise your foot off the floor and flex it outwards. Then draw large circles in the air by moving only your ankles.

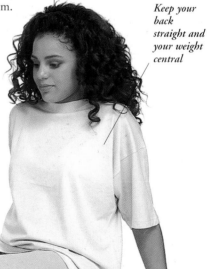

YOUR PELVIC FLOOR

The pelvic floor muscles form a funnel that supports the uterus, bowel and bladder, and serve to close the entrances to the vagina, rectum and urethra.

During pregnancy, an increase in progesterone causes the muscles to soften and relax. To counter this there is an exercise you can do to keep the pelvic floor well-toned.

Pull in and tense the muscles around your vagina and anus, as if you were stopping the flow of urine. Hold as long as you can without straining. Relax. Repeat as often as possible each day.

You should begin this exercise again as soon as you can after delivery to minimize the risk of prolapse. Early exercise will tone up the vagina for sexual intercourse too. If possible, make this exercise part of your daily routine.

EXERCISES FOR THE BODY

By performing exercises for your whole body, you will relieve the strain caused by your extra weight and strengthen important muscles. Also, if you learn to move your pelvis easily during pregnancy, you will be better able to find the most comfortable position during labour. A major proponent of active birth, Janet Balaskas, specializes in prenatal exercises using modified yoga positions. Some of her suggestions are shown here.

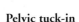
Make sure your back is straight

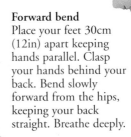
Raise your arms as high as you can

Forward bend
Place your feet 30cm (12in) apart keeping hands parallel. Clasp your hands behind your back. Bend slowly forward from the hips, keeping your back straight. Breathe deeply.

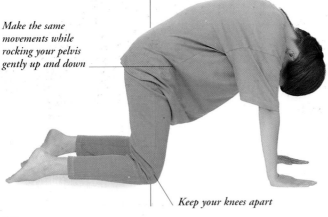

Make the same movements while rocking your pelvis gently up and down

Keep your knees apart

Pelvic tuck-in
Kneel down on all fours with your knees about 30cm (12in) apart. Clench your buttock muscles and tuck in your pelvis so that your back arches upwards into a hump. Hold this position for a few seconds, and then release, making sure you do not let your back sink downwards. Repeat this manoeuvre several times.

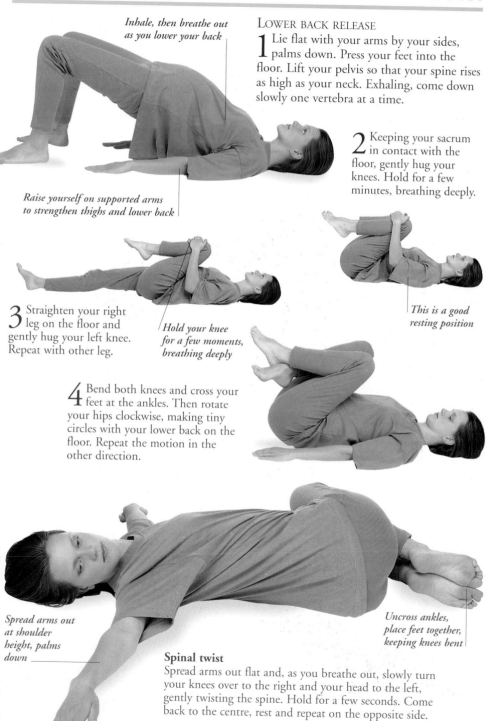

Inhale, then breathe out as you lower your back

LOWER BACK RELEASE

1 Lie flat with your arms by your sides, palms down. Press your feet into the floor. Lift your pelvis so that your spine rises as high as your neck. Exhaling, come down slowly one vertebra at a time.

2 Keeping your sacrum in contact with the floor, gently hug your knees. Hold for a few minutes, breathing deeply.

Raise yourself on supported arms to strengthen thighs and lower back

3 Straighten your right leg on the floor and gently hug your left knee. Repeat with other leg.

Hold your knee for a few moments, breathing deeply

This is a good resting position

4 Bend both knees and cross your feet at the ankles. Then rotate your hips clockwise, making tiny circles with your lower back on the floor. Repeat the motion in the other direction.

Spread arms out at shoulder height, palms down

Uncross ankles, place feet together, keeping knees bent

Spinal twist

Spread arms out flat and, as you breathe out, slowly turn your knees over to the right and your head to the left, gently twisting the spine. Hold for a few seconds. Come back to the centre, rest and repeat on the opposite side.

SHAPING UP FOR LABOUR

You may have a more comfortable experience in labour if you have prepared your body in advance. Some women find it easier to give birth in the squatting position, and practising tailor sitting will strengthen your thigh muscles, increase circulation to your pelvis, make the joints more supple, and stretch and help relax your perineum. After any bout of exercise, spend 20–30 minutes relaxing. Relaxation techniques are also beneficial in labour, when tension can increase the pain.

Tailor sitting
Sit on the floor and, making sure your back is straight, bend your knees and bring the soles of your feet together, then pull them towards your body. Open out your thighs and lower your knees towards the floor. Relax your shoulders.

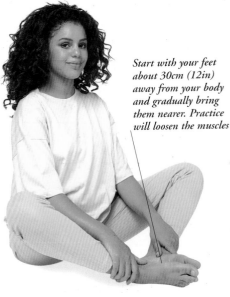

Start with your feet about 30cm (12in) away from your body and gradually bring them nearer. Practice will loosen the muscles

Squatting
Stand with your back straight and your feet apart. Squat down as low as you can. Linking hands, spread and hold your knees apart with your elbows. Try to keep your heels on the ground with your weight even. Hold this for as long as you can.

Squat to become flexible and to stretch and strengthen the thigh and back muscles

Relaxation
As your abdomen gets bigger you may find it more comfortable to lie on your side. Bend your upper arm and leg upwards and place a pillow under this knee; keep your lower leg straight.

Pressure on the major blood vessels and the abdomen is alleviated by lying in this way

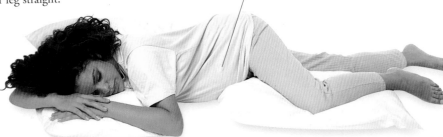

TAKING CARE OF YOURSELF

The happier and healthier you are, the better it is for your baby's development and the more you will enjoy your pregnancy. Relaxation, looking good and feeling on top of things are all-important – especially during this time when you may worry about your changing appearance. Whatever you consume can affect your unborn baby, so it is sensible to eat wisely and avoid anything that is potentially harmful. Emotional changes due to fluctuating hormones may bring any doubts and fears to the surface but this is a natural part of becoming a mother. Your constant awareness of your unborn baby is the first stage in bonding with her.

MASSAGE AIDS

Massage is very sensual – using a variety of lovely smells, textures and pressures can add greatly to the experience. To avoid breaking the rhythm, have everything ready before beginning the massage.

• *Scented oils are wonderful to help your hands glide over the skin, and leave it soft and smooth. Their fragrance will add to the atmosphere, making each occasion special.*

• *Feathers, velvet, silk and other soft-textured materials can be rubbed over the skin to leave it tingling.*

• *Warm, fluffy towels are comforting and ideal for keeping you warm.*

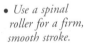

• *Use a spinal roller for a firm, smooth stroke.*

• *A soft bristle hairbrush used to brush the hair with light strokes is very soothing and relaxing.*

GENTLE MASSAGE FOR RELAXATION

A massage, whether given by a partner or one that you give yourself, is an ideal way to relax and unwind. It stimulates the nerve endings in your skin, improves your circulation, and soothes tired muscles, creating an overall sense of peace and well-being.

THE SOOTHING TOUCH

Use a good-quality massage oil (almond or vegetable oils are best) to reduce the friction between hands and skin and make the massage more pleasurable. Create a comfortable atmosphere: dim the lighting and have pillows or cushions around and underneath yourself. In the later months, you may find it more comfortable to lie on your side supported by pillows, or to sit astride a chair.

Apart from your back, you can massage most parts of your body yourself. Massage your abdomen, hips and thighs with the palms of your hands, using a smooth, circular motion. Work clockwise around each breast, gently kneading from the base towards the nipple.

SELF-MASSAGE

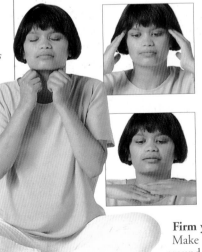

Soothe your forehead
Place your fingertips on your forehead and the heels of your hands on your chin. Gently draw your hands apart towards your temples.

Tone your chin
Stimulate the blood circulation under your chin with brisk but gentle slapping movements using the back of both hands.

Firm your neck
Make gentle pinching movements around your jawbone. Softly squeeze the skin between your thumb and the knuckles of your index finger.

If you are to be massaged by a partner or a friend, make sure the masseur's hands are warm before starting the massage, and he or she should remove any rings, bracelets or watches that may scratch or jangle. When you are both in comfortable positions, take a few deep breaths to help you relax. The massage should begin gently and the pressure gradually increase only if it is comfortable for you. Here are a few ideas to try:

Circling   Use the palms of both hands simultaneously to make circling strokes in the same direction away from the spine. Lighten the pressure when massaging over the abdomen and breasts.

Effleurage   Make light, feathery, circular movements with the fingertips as though tickling the skin. This can be done all over the abdomen during pregnancy.

Gliding   Place the palms of both hands on either side of the sacrum in the back, with the fingers towards the head. Push the hands up towards the shoulders, without letting the weight of the body onto the hands. Slowly glide back to the starting point.

ESSENTIAL OILS

Aromatic oils can greatly enhance your massage, helping you feel relaxed and refreshed. Their diverse scents may also conjure up wonderful images or moods.

These oils are distilled from flowers, trees and herbs, and are said to have therapeutic qualities. Lavender oil, for example, relieves headaches and insomnia, and jasmine helps treat postnatal depression. Always blend essential oils with a light carrier oil such as almond.

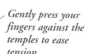

MASSAGE BY A PARTNER

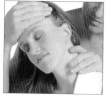

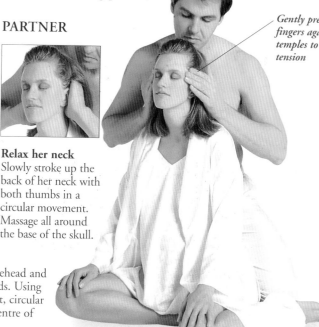

Gently press your fingers against the temples to ease tension

Support her head
Kneel behind her to massage her neck muscles. Gently turn her head, while keeping it well supported.

Relax her neck
Slowly stroke up the back of her neck with both thumbs in a circular movement. Massage all around the base of the skull.

Stroke her brow
Gently massage her forehead and temples with both hands. Using your fingers, make light, circular movements from the centre of her forehead outwards.

41

EMOTIONAL CHANGES

It is not only your body that alters during pregnancy, your emotions will fluctuate rapidly and you may experience depths of emotion that you have never had before. It is important to recognize that you will feel upset from time to time, that all pregnant women do, and that there are things you can do that will help with your mood swings.

HORMONAL CHANGES

Enormous changes occur in your body during pregnancy and, because of this, your mood is likely to alter frequently. It is not unusual to find yourself becoming hypercritical and irritable, your reactions to minor events may be exaggerated, you may feel unsure of yourself and panicky sometimes, and you may even have bouts of depression and crying.

It is normal to feel all of these things, because you are less in control of your feelings than usual. At work, you may have to struggle to preserve a veneer of calm. This effort will definitely pay off, especially if you plan to return to your job after the birth of your baby.

CHANGING BODY SHAPE

Under normal circumstances, it takes some time to adjust to a change in body image, such as losing or gaining a large amount of weight. In pregnancy you are not given time to adjust to the shape of your body, and you may feel strange about it. You may also worry that you are putting on too much weight and that you will become fat and unattractive during or after pregnancy.

Thinking of pregnant women as fat, and therefore ugly, is essentially an Anglo-Saxon attitude: many other cultures regard pregnant women as sensuous and beautiful. Instead of viewing your increasing curves with despair, think of them as a re-affirmation of life; see the roundness as ripeness, and glory in the fertility of your body. Feel confident and proud of your pregnant shape.

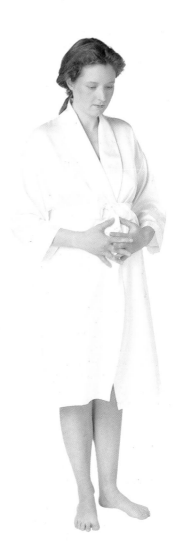

Your changing shape
As you get larger, a positive attitude to your appearance is important because it will help you stay cheerful.

CONFLICTING FEELINGS

Even with the most positive attitudes about pregnancy it is normal to have conflicting feelings. One moment you are thrilled at the prospect of a new baby, the next minute you are terrified of your new responsibilities. Becoming a parent is a time of reassessment and change, of expressing and discussing your worries and fears.

The first and most important psychological task you have is to accept the pregnancy. This may sound obvious but there are women who unwisely go through the early months of pregnancy giving it as little thought as possible, which is especially easy until the baby begins to show. You and the baby's father have to come to terms with the pregnancy and begin to think about the reality – especially if, until now, your thoughts about a baby and parenthood have probably all been in soft focus, a pastel picture of a loving threesome.

Conflicting feelings are sure to surface once you begin to accept the pending realities of responsibility and loss of freedom. Let me reassure you that it's normal to feel this way and you shouldn't worry about it. It means that you are genuinely coming to terms with the situation. You won't go into shock as some people do when they suddenly have to face all this on the baby's arrival.

FEARS

You may be worried about labour – whether you will be able to cope with the pain, whether you will scream or defecate, lose control, or need an episiotomy or emergency Caesarean. Most women worry about these things, but there's really no need. Labour is usually straightforward and how you behave will be of little or no consequence. You may be surprised at how calm you are or you may not be calm at all, and that's okay too. Just remember that your birth attendants have seen it all before, so there is nothing to feel embarrassed about.

You may worry about how good a parent you'll be, whether you will hurt or harm your baby, or not care for her properly. These kinds of feelings are quite common and represent legitimate fears. Like many other modern women, you probably do not know much about baby care and are worried about doing a good job. The answer is to get some hands-on experience – handle and care for a newborn baby if you can. Perhaps you could babysit for a friend's baby, or spend some time with her. If you change and feed her, you will probably gain confidence. Try to get these fears into perspective – you probably had similar worries about starting a new job.

WILL MY MOOD AFFECT MY BABY?

You may worry that your fluctuating emotional changes will somehow adversely affect your unborn baby.

Although your baby reacts to your moods, such as kicking when you are angry or upset, your changeable emotions appear to have no detrimental effect on your baby (see p. 47).

On the other hand, your baby really enjoys your good moods – your excitement, your happiness and your elation. When you feel good, your baby feels good. When you're relaxed, your baby is also tranquil.

If some activity makes you content and happy, do as much of it as you can and share the feeling with your baby.

WHAT DO MY DREAMS MEAN?

Dreams may become more frequent, and even frightening, in the last trimester. There are many common themes reported by pregnant women and all express deep feelings and concerns that are entirely natural.

Dreams about losing the baby are usually an expression of fear about miscarrying or having a stillborn baby. Such dreams may be a psychological preparation for a possible unwanted outcome and also a way of bringing these feelings to the surface. In a way, they act as a release for your anxieties.

KEEPING A DIARY

Keeping a diary at any time of your life can give you insights about yourself that you might not normally take the time to consider.

It is a place where you can express those thoughts and feelings that you may not want to share, and where you can focus on yourself. Your child may also enjoy reading it – especially when she is pregnant.

Pregnancy journal
As well as providing a place to note your progress, keeping a journal means that you will have a cherished record of this special time in your life to look back on.

SUPERSTITIONS

It is possible that you may be more superstitious than normal. Superstition and old wives' tales were, in the past, ways of explaining an inexplicable world. With the excellent medical care now available, your chances of having an imperfect child are low, and what you might interpret as a bad omen certainly does not mean that anything will go wrong with your baby.

COPING WITH EMOTIONAL CHANGES

Try to see the emotional turmoil you are experiencing as a positive force as you adjust to being pregnant and becoming a mother. Don't imagine that having second thoughts or fears means that you've made a mistake. You're tossing this around in your head the way one wrestles with any big life decision. Yet social conditioning makes us feel guilty if we don't walk around with a madonna-like expression. That is absurd. Being pregnant isn't all fun. Accepting the reality is the best thing you can do for yourself and your child.

Spend time daydreaming Imagining and thinking about your baby helps you to form a relationship with her even before she is born, and you shouldn't feel silly if you find that you spend a couple of hours doing nothing but thinking about the baby. Making that connection with the tiny person growing inside you is the first step in accepting your child.

Consider your parents Becoming a grandparent can often be viewed as being synonymous with becoming old, and can be unsettling for a person who perhaps feels only just middle-aged. Try to be understanding and loving, include them in your pregnancy, share your feelings with them.

Confront your isolation It is quite common for a pregnant woman to feel isolated nowadays. Many women are postponing having children, and some are deciding against it altogether. You may find that you are the first in your social circle to start a family, and that you don't know any other pregnant women or fully fledged mothers. It can be lonely. If so, look for people to whom you can talk – join parent groups, approach other pregnant women in your childbirth classes, and ask your friends or family if they know any pregnant women whom you could get to know. These friendships may provide support long after your baby is born. Don't forget your partner either – include him and expand your social circle together.

Communicate Wanting to talk and share what you are feeling and thinking during your pregnancy is natural. Your partner is the logical first choice, and there are bound to be things that he would like to talk about: worries that he may have refrained from discussing with you because he thought that he might upset you, or you might think him silly, or because you were too busy, or too tired. Keep talking. You need each other more now than ever before. Denying or ignoring your fears and feelings won't make them go away. Suppressed feelings have a very nasty way of festering and then surfacing when you are least equipped to deal with them, thus becoming full-blown problems.

COPING WITH MATERIAL CHANGES

Everyday difficulties that you would normally deal with quite calmly can turn into dramas during pregnancy. Keep a level head, and try not to overreact.

Finances One of the major causes of marital strife, financial problems can become especially troubling during pregnancy. You may find it difficult to cope with an inevitable reduction in income, even if you plan to return to work, but remember that you are in this together. Work out before the birth how you will live on your income once the baby has arrived.

Housing Moving or expanding your home may be something that you are forced to consider – perhaps you need the extra space, or it may be because of the lack of facilities in your area. This can be stressful, and tends to be worse when you are expecting. If you must move – and many couples do, although it's not really recommended from a physical standpoint – do it before your pregnancy is too advanced.

GRANDPARENTS

A new baby means a new role not only for you but possibly also for your parents.

While they will, no doubt, revel in their roles as doting grandparents once the baby is born, when you first tell them the glad tidings they may feel they are still too young. Their ambiguous response is natural – their lives are changing too.

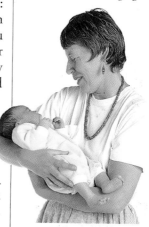

A source of help
Even before the baby is born, your parents can often be invaluable sources of information, expertise and reassurance – they have been through it all themselves.

GETTING IN TOUCH WITH YOUR BABY

WHAT YOU CAN DO

Communication can begin early on. What you say, do, think or experience, and the way you move may be transmitted to your baby.

Talk and sing *Get in the habit of talking out loud to your baby, and singing to her whenever possible. Some children have recognized lullabies that were played to them while they were still in the uterus.*

Touching *Stroking your baby through your abdominal wall is another way of getting in touch and will usually quieten her. This may continue after she is born. In the final months you may be able to distinguish the shape of a foot or hand through your skin.*

Thinking *Be aware of your baby. Think positive, happy thoughts about her. If you are upset about something, don't shut her out.*

Moving *Try to move in a relaxed manner whenever you can. The gentle movement of your body as you walk soothes her. Rocking and swinging will remain a favourite relaxing activity after she is born.*

Emotions *When you feel happy and excited, so does your baby. When you feel depressed, so does she – so reassure her that you still love her. Share feelings with her consciously.*

A constant awareness of your unborn baby is a first stage in bonding with her and ensuring a good future relationship. Getting in touch means that you are aware of what's best for your baby's physical and emotional health.

WHAT YOUR BABY EXPERIENCES

While she is still in your uterus, your baby feels, hears, sees, tastes, responds and even learns and remembers. She is not, contrary to decades of medical opinion, an inert, unformed, blank personality. She has firm likes and dislikes. She enjoys soothing voices, simple music with a single melody line (lullabies, flute music), rhythmic movements, and feeling you stroke her through your abdomen. Her dislikes include strident voices; music with an insistent beat (hard rock); strong, flashing lights; rapid, jerky movements; and being cramped when you sit or lie in an awkward position.

Sight Although your baby is shielded by the walls of your uterus and abdomen, light that is sufficiently strong can get through to her; for instance, she can detect sunlight if you are sunbathing. What she sees is probably just a reddish glow, but from about the fourth month, she will respond to it, usually by turning away if it is too bright. The limits of her sight at birth (she will be able to see faces within 20–25cm [8–10in] of her own) may be a consequence of the parameters of her "home" before birth.

Sound Your baby's sense of hearing develops at about the third month, and by midterm she is able to respond to sounds from the outside world (see above). The amniotic fluid in which she is suspended conducts sound well, although what she hears will be muffled in the same way that sounds are when you are under water. She is also able to distinguish the emotional tone of voices and moves her body in rhythm to your speech, so she will be soothed if you use a soft, reassuring tone.

The sound of your heartbeat is a continual presence in her world and this seems to be something that will have a profound influence on her. One study has found that when newborn babies were played a tape of maternal heart sounds, they gained more weight and slept better than a control group who did not hear the tape.

A MOTHER'S INFLUENCE

The unborn baby first experiences the world through her mother. Your baby experiences not only external stimuli (see above), but also your feelings, because our different emotions trigger the release of certain chemicals into our bloodstream – anger releases adrenaline, fear releases cholamines, elation releases endorphins. These chemicals pass across the placenta to your baby within seconds of you experiencing that particular emotion.

Babies dislike being exposed to prolonged levels of negative maternal emotions, such as anger, anxiety or fear. However, short periods of intense anxiety or anger (caused by a missing child or an argument with your partner, for example), do not appear to have any long-term negative effect on an unborn child. In fact, they may even be beneficial since they may help her to begin to develop the ability to cope with future stressful situations. On the other hand, research indicates that long-term festering anger or anxiety, such as you might experience in an unsatisfactory, unsupportive relationship or poor social conditions, can have detrimental effects on your baby. These effects appear to include a problematic birth, a low birthweight, being a colicky baby, and future learning problems. However, studies have found that long-term negative maternal emotions appear to have far less effect on the baby if the mother feels generally happy and positive about being pregnant.

A FATHER'S INFLUENCE

As the expectant father, you are the second most important factor in your unborn baby's life. Your attitude towards your partner, the pregnancy and your child is crucial. If you are happy and looking forward to your newborn, your partner is much more likely to be happy and to enjoy her pregnancy. This, in turn, means that your baby is much more likely to be a contented, healthy child. In addition, you should talk directly to your unborn baby as often as possible because research has shown that newborn babies can recognize the voices of their fathers and their mothers.

MAKE-UP TIPS

Pregnancy can change the tone and colour of your skin and you may want to adjust your make-up to counteract the effects.

Fine lines or wrinkles *These will become more accentuated if your skin becomes drier than usual, so stop using products that make them look more obvious; shiny or glittering eye shadows, heavy foundations and coloured powders will make them more prominent.*

Extra greasy skin *To combat this, use an astringent lotion, oil-free foundation, and dust with translucent powder.*

Extra dry skin *This is very rare in pregnancy, but if your skin becomes so dry that it flakes, you should avoid using make-up but continue to moisturize it well. If you must wear make-up, use an oil-based foundation and powder to help to slow water loss. Thick, creamy moisturizers will also act as a barrier to water loss on dry patches.*

High colour and spider veins *Stipple a thin, light coat of a neutral matt foundation that is free of any pink on to your cheeks. When dry, cover with your regular foundation and a transparent powder.*

Dark circles *Under your eyes, over a thin layer of foundation, lightly dab on a cover-up cream and leave to dry. Cover with another thin layer of foundation and blend carefully. Finish with a dusting of transparent powder.*

YOUR BODY

The pregnancy hormones bring about changes to almost every part of your body, including your skin, hair, teeth and gums. Moreover, your enlarging abdomen will affect your posture, possibly causing backache and fatigue, so it is important to look after your body and pay particular attention to the way you stand or move (see p. 50).

SKIN

Your skin will probably "bloom" during pregnancy because the hormones encourage it to retain moisture that plumps it out, making it more supple, less oily and less prone to spots. The extra blood circulating round your body will also cause your skin to glow. However, the opposite can sometimes happen. Red patches may enlarge, acne may worsen, areas may become dry and scaly, and you may notice deeper pigmentation across your face, particularly if you have freckles.

Skin care If your skin is drier during pregnancy, avoid using soap because it removes the natural oils from the skin. Try using baby lotion, or glycerine-based soap and body wash instead. Always use oils in the bath to minimize the dehydrating effects of hard water, and do not lie in a bath for long because prolonged contact with water particularly dehydrates the skin. Using make-up is good for your morale, and can also act as a moisturizer for the skin as it prevents water loss (see column, left).

Skin pigmentation Nearly all pregnant woman are affected by deeper pigmentation, especially in the areas that are pigmented to begin with, for example, freckles, moles and the areolae of the breasts. Your genitalia, the skin of the inner sides of the thighs, under your eyes and in your armpits may become darker too.

A dark line, called the *linea nigra*, often appears down the centre of your stomach. It marks the division of your abdominal muscles, which separate slightly to accommodate your expanding uterus.

After birth, the *linea nigra* and the areolae usually remain darker for some time, but all pigmentation will gradually fade and disappear. Sunlight intensifies all areas of skin that are already pigmented, and many women find that they tan more easily during pregnancy. Keep your skin covered up in hot sun, or use a sun block, especially on the face and delicate areas such as your nipples.

Chloasma This is a type of pigmentation, also called the mask of pregnancy, which appears as brown patches on the bridge of the nose, cheeks and neck. The only way to cope with chloasma is to camouflage it with a blemish stick or the cover-up cosmetics that are used for birthmarks. Never try to bleach out the pigment; the patches will begin to fade within three months of labour. Some black women develop patches of paler skin (vitiligo) on their faces and necks. These also usually disappear after delivery and can be camouflaged during pregnancy.

Spider veins In pregnancy, all the blood vessels become sensitive – rapidly dilating when you are hot, and constricting quickly when you are cold. Consequently, tiny broken blood vessels called spider veins may appear on your face, particularly on your cheeks. Do not worry; these should disappear altogether within three months.

Pimples If your skin has a tendency to become spotty before periods, you may get pimples now, particularly in the first trimester when the pregnancy hormones stimulating the sebaceous glands in the skin have not yet settled down. Try to keep your skin as clean as possible, and use a cleanser two or three times a day to prevent spots altogether. If a spot appears, do not squeeze it but apply a tiny smear of antiseptic cream.

Stretch marks About 90 percent of pregnant women get stretch marks. These usually appear across the stomach, although they can also affect the thighs, hips, breasts and the upper arms. Nothing you can apply to the skin (including oil), and nothing you eat will prevent stretch marks because they are due to the breakdown of protein in the skin by the high levels of pregnancy hormones. Gradual weight gain should allow the skin to stretch without thinning, although some women are blessed with more elastic skin than others. While the reddish streaks look prominent during pregnancy, after delivery they become paler until they are faint silvery streaks that are barely noticeable.

YOUR HAIR

During pregnancy, it is very common for the hair to change in quality, quantity and manageability.

The high levels of hormones arrest the usual cycle of hair growth and loss. Usually, some hair grows and some is lost every day. In pregnancy, however, the cycle is arrested in the growth phase.

After delivery, the growth cycle passes into a resting phase when hair can be shed at an alarming rate. Hair loss can go on for up to two years but rest assured, it will stop – pregnancy never causes baldness. This hair is simply what you would normally have lost throughout the nine months of pregnancy.

Body and facial hair may also increase in quantity and may even darken in colour.

YOUR TEETH

You will be more susceptible than normal to gum problems owing to the high level of progesterone, which softens all of your body's tissues.

The tiny capillaries around the gum margin often bleed easily. A balanced diet with sufficient calcium and first-class protein, along with a good supply of vitamins B, C and D, helps prevent teeth and gum problems. You should see your dentist at least once during your pregnancy but be sure to tell him or her that you are pregnant because you should avoid X-rays.

49

MAINTAINING GOOD POSTURE

Adopting and maintaining a good posture will help you to minimize the backache and fatigue that can easily arise as your pregnancy advances.

Bad posture is a common problem in pregnancy. It is caused by the increasing weight of your baby. Your enlarging abdomen thrusts your centre of gravity forward, and to balance this you tend to arch your back backwards, putting your back muscles under constant strain – hence backache.

When you are standing, sitting, or walking with the correct posture, your neck and back will be in a straight line.

AVOIDING PROBLEMS

The pregnancy hormones stretch and soften your ligaments, particularly in the lower back, making them more vulnerable to strain. However, with a little care you can avoid the unnecessary problems and fatigue that many women suffer during pregnancy.

PROTECT YOUR BACK

Don't bend down
When you are doing household chores or working in the garden and you need to work on something at floor level, sit or kneel to bring it within easy reach. Whenever possible, avoid bending or stooping.

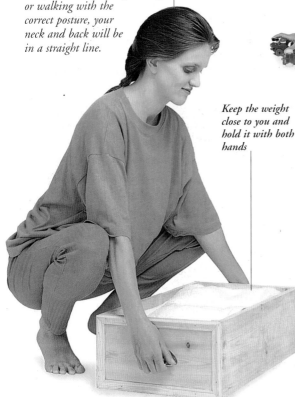

Keep the weight close to you and hold it with both hands

Sit back on your heels, but try to avoid making your legs go numb

Lifting and carrying
To lift something from the floor, reach down to it by bending your knees, keeping your back as straight as you can. When you pick it up, hold it close in to your body, and lift it by straightening your legs, so that you use the strength of your leg and thigh muscles to do the actual lifting. Never struggle to lift objects that are too heavy – get someone to help you. Don't try lifting heavy things to or from high shelves or upwards. If you are carrying heavy bags, try to divide the weight equally between both hands.

Getting up

When you have been lying down in bed or on the floor, for instance if you have been exercising, get up in easy stages. First, turn on to your side (see below), then use your hands to support yourself as you move yourself into a kneeling position (see top right). From there, keeping your back straight and using the strength of your thigh muscles, push yourself up into a sitting position. From here you can stand up without straining your abdomen.

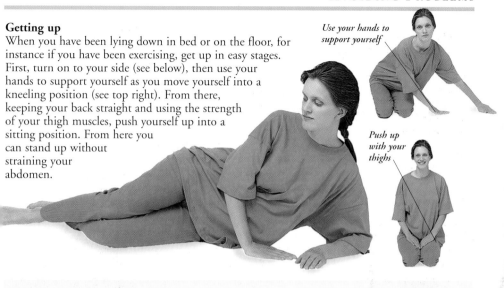

Use your hands to support yourself

Push up with your thighs

SKIN AND NAIL PROBLEMS

POSSIBLE PROBLEMS	WHAT TO DO
Itching or chafed skin The skin of your extended abdomen may become quite itchy, and the area between your thighs may become a little chafed.	Massage your skin with baby lotion to stimulate the blood supply and ease irritation. Keep the thigh area dry; dust with powder and wear cotton underwear. If the area becomes red and sore, apply zinc cream.
Rashes These are not uncommon in the groin and under the breasts, and are a result of excess weight gain and sweat that accumulates in the skin folds. Poor hygiene will increase the risk.	Keep your groin area and the skin under your breasts clean, and apply calamine or other drying lotion. Take care to keep your weight gain under control. Wear a firm, supporting bra to hold up the breasts.
Pigmentation Many women find that their skin pigmentation alters when they are pregnant; this particularly affects darker areas such as freckles, moles and the areolae of the breasts.	Use a sun block to protect your skin from the ultraviolet rays in sunlight. The pigmentation effects will disappear after the birth.
Brittle nails Your fingernails will grow faster than usual during pregnancy, but they may also become brittle and split or break more easily than they did before you became pregnant.	Keep your nails short, and wear protective gloves for housework and gardening.

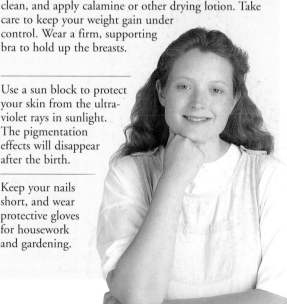

MATERNITY WEAR

Comfort is the watchword during pregnancy as far as clothes are concerned. A good support bra is an essential, and as your size increases, try to stay one step ahead – there's nothing more demoralizing than feeling constricted and too big for your clothes. You'll find that because the blood is circulating round your body at a faster rate, you'll probably be warmer than normal during pregnancy; so choose light and loose-fitting clothes. Feet and legs tend to swell, particularly towards the end of the pregnancy, so you'll probably have to buy a larger size in footwear and hosiery.

CLOTHES

Pregnancy doesn't have to mean lots of expensive maternity clothes. Buy a few basics, such as a pair of maternity jeans with an expandable front panel, a selection of properly fitted maternity bras (see opposite), some maternity cotton or wool tights and leggings with expandable gussets, and one or two pretty maternity dresses for special occasions. Add to these some drawstring trousers and man-size tops and jumpers – all of which can be worn when you are no longer pregnant. Avoid clothes made of synthetic fabrics whenever you can as they're not as comfortable as natural fabrics. Stretch fabrics, for example, can become unpleasantly clingy and tight; polyester tends to trap moisture, causing discomfort in hot weather.

Work clothes Depending on where you work, you may be able to get away with wearing smarter versions of your casual wear, such as maternity trousers with an elegant top or a loose cotton skirt with a crisp cotton blouse. However, if you work in an environment where formal clothes are worn, you may have to invest in higher-priced maternity suits, or perhaps ordinary long-line jackets, large-size skirts and blouses, and drop-waist dresses may suffice. If you wear a uniform, make sure that you tell your employers as soon as you know that you are pregnant, as they may be able to offer you a larger size if they have sufficient notice. It is best to wear flat shoes at work, even if you normally wear heels, especially if you have to stand all day.

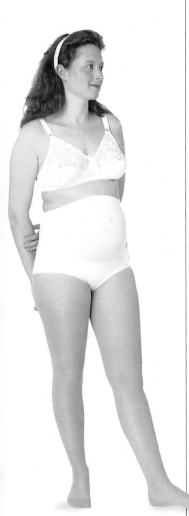

Maternity underwear
A pregnancy bra and girdle can be invaluable for your comfort during pregnancy – and for your figure afterwards.

SHOES

The bigger you get, the more unstable you become, so it's a good idea to wear flat or low-heeled, comfortable, easy-fitting shoes. They should give your feet good support, be sufficiently roomy, and preferably have a non-slip sole for safety. Trainers fulfil all the criteria, and if possible choose a pair with a Velcro fastening because later in pregnancy it may be difficult for you to bend down to do up the laces. There are lots of smart, flat shoes available that are versatile and durable. Your feet will swell during pregnancy, so choose a size bigger than normal, and avoid anything with a heel.

UNDERWEAR

Maternity bra This is one item that is essential in pregnancy. Your breasts may enlarge substantially, particularly during the first three months, and if you don't support them, they are likely to sag later. This is because the sling of fibrous tissue to which they are attached can never regain its former shape once it is overstretched. A well-fitting support bra will help to prevent stretching in the first place.

When you buy a bra, it is best to have it properly fitted. A store specializing in maternity clothes or lingerie, or a large department store, is likely to have specially trained staff. Make sure that the bra of your choice gives you good support with a deep band underneath the cups and wide shoulder straps that won't cut into your skin. Fastening should be adjustable for comfort, so back-fastening bras may be better than front-fastening. Only buy a couple of bras to begin with as your breasts will continue to grow, and you'll have to get larger sizes later in pregnancy. If your breasts become very big it is a good idea to wear a light bra in bed at night to give them extra support. Just before your due date buy a few front-opening feeding bras and breast pads to make breastfeeding easier. These can be bought in any maternity shop or department store.

Girdles Wearing a maternity girdle during the second and third trimester will give you much-needed support – especially if you are expecting more than one baby. By relieving the strain, a girdle can also help prevent backache.

HOSIERY

Socks *These should be made of cotton or wool and be loose-fitting; synthetic materials don't give and can cut really deeply into swollen feet. In addition, they don't allow your sweat to evaporate, so the skin may become waterlogged and soft. Avoid knee-high socks because these can form a restricting band around the top of your calf, encouraging varicose veins (see p. 68).*

Tights *Maternity tights (even sheer ones) can give a lot of support and help prevent aching legs. There are many different types available in a variety of colours. You will find them in maternity shops and most department stores.*

Stockings *If you find that you suffer from severe thrush (a common complaint in pregnancy), you may prefer to wear stockings rather than tights. Support stockings, or ones containing a high percentage of lycra, will probably be the most comfortable, although they obviously don't offer the same amount of support as maternity tights. A suspender belt can be more comfortable if it fits on your hips under your belly, so choose one that is big enough and shorten the straps if necessary.*

There are a few minor adjustments that you can make to your normal working lifestyle that will make your day more comfortable.

Put your feet up *Sit down as much as possible, and put your feet up whenever you can. At the office, convert a piece of furniture such as an overturned bin, or an extended drawer into a foot stool.*

Relaxation exercises *Practise a few simple neck, shoulder, pelvic and foot exercises as often as possible when at work. These will release any tension, and help to improve your circulation.*

Practise squatting *Use the squatting position whenever you have to bend down, or if there is no chair available. You will strengthen your thighs, and prepare yourself to use this position at the delivery.*

Eat well *Keep a supply of nutritious snacks available (see p. 24). Although you may still have feelings of nausea, your urge for food may strike at inconvenient moments. A wholemeal biscuit or cracker, and a glass of semi-skimmed milk will be filling, and may help relieve attacks of nausea.*

Take it easy *In general, you should just try to take things more slowly. Stop whenever you feel fatigued and try to get some rest every afternoon or in the early evening.*

A WORKING PREGNANCY

Pregnancy brings with it a variety of physical changes and discomforts but continuing to work can give you the psychological benefit of affirming that pregnancy is a normal state, not an illness. Working also enables you to maintain this important and stable aspect of your life at a time when you may be feeling disorientated by the changes created by your pregnancy.

YOUR RIGHTS AT WORK

Most employers will be keen to co-operate with your wish to carry on working during and after your pregnancy, provided that you keep them informed (in writing) of when you plan to stop work before your baby is born and when you plan to resume it afterwards (see below).

Protect your job Discuss with your employer or your trade union representative your entitlements concerning maternity leave and pay. By law you are allowed time off with pay in order to attend your antenatal check-ups, and this also includes relaxation classes.

Protect your health If there is the possibility of your work causing harm to your baby, for example if X-rays or heavy lifting fall within your area of responsibility, your employer should find you an alternative job while you are pregnant, provided that you have worked with the company for an adequate period.

ADAPTING YOUR ROUTINE

Coping with fatigue while working is an ever-present necessity when you are pregnant. Bouts of morning sickness, particularly in early pregnancy, can make the situation even more difficult. As your pregnancy progresses, the weight you're carrying will cause you to feel that even walking is hard work, so avoid working long hours that leave you feeling exhausted. Over-tiredness will exacerbate any nausea or backache, and you could also find yourself losing concentration. Added to this is the stress of travelling to and from your job which, especially if you use public transport during the busy times, can be very wearing. However, if this is your situation, the solution may be to find out what you can alter during pregnancy.

You may, for example, be able to change the times you start and finish work to avoid travelling in the rush hour. If you have to do a lot of standing or walking at work, see whether you can take up a more sedentary role for the time being.

Take it easy Don't push yourself too hard in other areas of your life. Let domestic priorities slide by adopting a more lenient attitude towards household chores. Your health and that of your baby are far more important than having an immaculate house. Rest and relaxation are vital during pregnancy and you should allow yourself enough free time for a nap, an exercise routine and possibly a massage.

Ask for help At home, if you don't have help with the cooking and cleaning, ask your partner to assist. Maybe you could leave most of the chores until the weekend and do them together. Let your work colleagues know you're pregnant early on so that they are more likely to be understanding of your condition with its mood swings, lack of energy and the need for a less stressful working day.

DECIDING WHEN TO STOP

Some women happily continue working until they are near their due date. However, most medical authorities believe that you should not work beyond the 32nd week. It is around this time that your heart, lungs and other vital organs have to work harder, and when a great deal of strain is placed on your spine, joints and muscles. You should get rest whenever possible, and that is often difficult if you continue working.

DECIDING WHEN TO RETURN

Once you have the baby, you may wish to go back to work under different conditions, and you will have to discuss this with your employer – preferably before you return. If there is a provision for part-time employment, or a phased return that allows you to be, in effect, a part-time worker for up to one year after your baby's birth, these are ideal solutions. You could also investigate job sharing, flexible hours, or working from home in a freelance capacity. If these options are not available, you will have to consider what full-time childcare you can find in your area (and the costs) before you decide on returning to work.

YOUR BABY'S SAFETY

Try to be aware of any hazards in your workplace that may potentially harm your baby (see p. 58). If you are worried, talk to your doctor and employer about the risks, and take steps to avoid them.

Many mothers working in an office environment are particularly concerned about exposure to radiation from copying machines and computer video display terminals. However, recent reports state that these very low levels of radiation will not harm the developing baby.

If you work in a smoking environment, find out whether it is possible for you to transfer to a smoke-free zone, at least while you are pregnant and after the birth until you have finished breastfeeding.

DRUGS AND YOUR BABY

Consult your doctor before taking any drug – whether it is prescription or non-prescription, and whenever you have to consult a doctor always say that you're pregnant.

It is best to avoid taking any medication during pregnancy unless your doctor determines that the benefit to you outweighs any risk to the fetus. The long-term effects of many drugs on the unborn child are still largely unknown. Other drugs have been proven to be hazardous to the fetus and should be completely avoided (see below).

AVOIDING HAZARDS

Many of our normal activities may pose dangers during pregnancy. Cleaning out cat litter at home, or contact with harmful chemicals at work, passive smoking while socializing, or having vaccinations for travelling may affect the development of the unborn baby and certain precautions should be taken.

AT HOME

Very few of us can move to a perfect environment while pregnant, but you should try to avoid handling raw meat, touching other people's pets and cleaning out litter trays, breathing in exhaust gases from cars, and working with pesticides in the garden. Alcohol, coffee, and teas containing caffeine are also best avoided. Most herbal teas are generally safe (although you should always check this; avoid raspberry leaf, which is said to trigger contractions). Choose organic ones to avoid the risk of pesticides.

Harmful chemicals You should limit your use of aerosol sprays in the home, and there are alternatives to most aerosols on the market today. Although many modern

HOW DRUGS CAN AFFECT YOUR BABY

DRUG	USE	EFFECTS ON THE FETUS
Amphetamines	Stimulants	May cause heart defects and blood diseases
Anabolic steroids	Body-building	Can have a masculinizing effect on a female fetus
Tetracycline	Treats acne	Can colour first and permanent teeth yellow
Streptomycin	Treats tuberculosis	Can cause deafness in infants
Antihistamines	Allergies/travel sickness	Some cause malformations
Anti-nausea drugs	Combat nausea	May cause malformations
Aspirin	Painkillers	Can cause problems with blood clotting
Diuretics	Rid body of excess fluid	Can cause fetal blood disorders
Narcotics (Codeine, etc.)	Painkillers	Addictive; baby may suffer withdrawal symptoms
Paracetamol	Reduces pain and fever	Large doses can damage baby's kidneys and liver
LSD, cannabis	For "fun"	Risk of chromosomal damage, and miscarriage
Sulphonamides	Treat infections	Can cause jaundice in the baby at birth

aerosols contain substances (other than CFCs) that have not been implicated in causing harm to the fetus or mother, my feeling is that we are all exposed to invisible sources of potentially harmful chemicals, and it's wise to take every possible precaution.

Avoid substances that give off vapours, such as glue and petrol, as they may be toxic and should never be inhaled, whether you are pregnant or not. Read the label of any material you use, and avoid those that are potentially harmful. Some examples are cleaning fluids, contact cement, creosote, volatile paint, lacquers, thinners, some glues and oven cleaner. Hair perms are apparently safe in pregnancy, but if you have fears about their long-term effects, I would advise you to wait until after the first three months, when the most crucial organs in your baby's body have formed.

Hot baths Saunas and hot whirlpools have been implicated in fetal abnormalities, particularly those of the baby's nervous system, in exactly the same way as fever. When your body is subjected to extreme heat over a lengthy period, you can become overheated and this may affect your baby. Avoid saunas and whirlpools, especially in the first trimester, and keep bath temperatures moderate.

Television rays Rays, even from colour television, have not been shown to form ionizing radiation. It is not harmful to sit within several feet of the screen, even for long periods. However, make sure you are sitting comfortably to avoid backache.

Immunizations Because your entire immune system is changing under the influence of your pregnancy and may be weakened, your responses to various immunizations can be unpredictable.

Your doctor will discuss with you any immunizations that are necessary if you have been exposed to infectious diseases or if you have to travel outside the UK. In general, vaccinations that are prepared using live viruses – including those for measles, rubella (German measles), mumps, and yellow fever vaccinations – are best avoided. It is recommended that women do not have the flu vaccine during pregnancy, unless there is an underlying high risk of heart or lung disease.

TOXOPLASMOSIS AND YOUR BABY

This is an organism that normally produces only mild flu-like symptoms in an adult, but it can seriously damage the unborn child.

During pregnancy it can cause fetal brain damage, blindness and is fatal in certain cases. The greatest danger is during the third trimester.

Toxoplasma is carried in the faeces of infected animals, especially cats, but most people contract it by eating under-cooked meat. About 80% of the population have had it and have developed antibodies, but the younger you are, the less likely you are to be immune. You can ask your doctor to do a blood test for this.

Guidelines to follow:
- *Don't eat raw or under-cooked meat, especially pork, poultry or steak. Cook meat to an internal temperature of at least 55°C/131°F – at which bacteria is killed.*

- *Don't feed raw meat to your pets. Keep their food bowls away from everything else. Wash hands after feeding.*

- *Don't garden in soil that has been used by cats for litter and always wear gloves when gardening.*

- *Don't stroke or kiss other people's pets (particularly cats).*

- *Empty your cat's litter tray or touch your dog's faeces only if it is unavoidable. Wear gloves or wash your hands thoroughly in mild disinfectant afterwards.*

YOUR RISK OF INFECTION

In the first 12 weeks of pregnancy, you must try to avoid contact with anyone, expecially a child, who has a high fever, even if the fever is not thought to be caused by rubella (see p. 11).

If you contract mumps in pregnancy it will run the same course as if you were not pregnant. There is a minimal but increased risk of miscarriage if you get the disease in the first 12 weeks of pregnancy. The mumps vaccine is not given during pregnancy because it is "live" and could adversely affect the fetus.

Chickenpox is an uncommon disease in adults and is thus uncommon in pregnancy. It can cause fetal malformations.

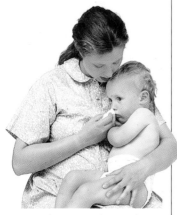

Infectious diseases
If you have small children there is obviously not much you can do to keep away from them. If you are a school teacher, be fairly strict about sending home any feverish child.

HAZARDS AT WORK

If you work outside the home, you may have many questions that have no simple answers: how safe is my workplace? Will the demands of my job put my pregnancy as risk? How long can I work?

If your job is strenuous, involving a lot of standing, walking, lifting or climbing, it may deprive you of the extra rest you need during pregnancy and aggravate fatigue. Your doctor may suggest that you reduce your work hours, transfer to less strenuous work or stop working several weeks before your estimated delivery date. In all circumstances, pregnant women must avoid those activities that expose them to physical danger, including some police work, motorcycle racing, competitive sports and so on.

Be alert to potentially harmful environmental factors and make sure that your employer transfers you to a working place or alternative job that does not contain hazards. Especially avoid the following:
- Anaesthetic gases (applicable to nurses, physicians, dentists and anaesthetists).
- Chemicals used in manufacturing and other industries – for example, lead, mercury, vinyl chloride, dry cleaning fluids, paint fumes and solvents.
- Close contact with animals that present a risk of toxoplasmosis (see p. 57).
- Exposure to infectious diseases (especially childhood illnesses such as rubella).
- Exposure to toxic wastes of any kind.
- Exposure to excessive levels of cigarette smoke, including passive smoking, for example in pubs and in offices that do not have smoking restrictions.
- Unacceptable levels of ionizing radiation (although these are now strictly monitored by government regulation).

It is generally accepted that day-to-day exposure to ultra-violet or infra-red radiation emitted by office equipment such as laser printers, copying machines and computer video display terminals is not dangerous to you or your baby. Therefore, if you work in a job presenting hazards no greater than those you encounter in daily life, you can usually work until close to your expected delivery date.

SOCIALIZING

Infections are caught from people with whom we come into contact. Although being pregnant doesn't mean that you should become a hermit, or wear a gauze mask when talking to people, it pays to be cautious – especially around children (see column, left), or adults who are running a raised temperature. Normal colds and flu will not harm your baby, but do your best to avoid running a fever. If your temperature goes very high, your doctor will advise what medications are safe (no aspirin in pregnancy) and using a damp sponge and a fan might help to cool the skin sufficiently. Don't take any cold or flu medicines that contain antihistamines.

TRAVELLING

There is absolutely no evidence that travel precipitates labour, or leads to miscarriage or any other complication of pregnancy. You should only be extra cautious if you have miscarried before, or have a history of premature labour. For long stays, ask your doctor for the name of an obstetrician in the area you are visiting and, in the last trimester, limit yourself to trips within 30 miles of home.

Trains Book a seat if possible, and make sure that it is not next to the buffet car as the smell may make you feel nauseous. Eat lightly to minimize motion sickness.

Cars Get out of the car at regular intervals and have a short walk to aid circulation. Always fasten your seat belt, but buckle it low, across your pelvis, and use a shoulder harness if you have one. You can do the driving as long as you are comfortable behind the wheel, but you must stop if you begin to feel cramped. Obviously, don't drive yourself to the hospital if you are in labour!

Air travel After your seventh month, air travel is not a good idea because of pressure changes in the cabin. If you must fly, check with the airline about whether they require a doctor's letter to let you on the plane after your seventh month. Do not fly in small private planes that have unpressurized cabins. If you sit over the wings or towards the front of the plane, you will feel less of the plane's motion.

TRAVELLING IN COMFORT

Bearing in mind a few important points when you are travelling could make it a more comfortable experience.

- *Leave more than enough time for your journey; allow yourself a comfortable margin between any connections you have to make.*

- *Travel in short bursts rather than for long stretches.*

- *Carry a drink, such as fruit juice or milk, in a flask.*

- *Take nutritious portable food, such as wholemeal crackers, fruit or vegetables, and nibbles including dried fruit, nuts and seeds.*

- *If nausea is a problem, carry glucose sweets to help prevent low blood sugar.*

FOREIGN TRAVEL

Take care when eating out that you follow the guidelines to avoid listeria and other food-related diseases (see p. 30). Drink bottled water if in doubt.

- *Check with your doctor which immunizations are safe (typhoid fever vaccinations, for example, could harm the baby but the cholera vaccine may not be harmful and you may need it to satisfy requirements in South East Asia).*

- *Rabies and tetanus vaccinations may be necessary, particularly if there is any indication of exposure.*

GETTING ENOUGH SLEEP

A good night's sleep is one of your top priorities in the late stages of pregnancy.

Aim to get eight hours of sleep a night, but you may suffer from irritating insomnia because, although your metabolism slows down at night, that of your baby does not. It keeps hammering away all through the night hours. If you cannot sleep, there are a number of ways in which you can alleviate the problem:

• A warm bath before going to bed is very relaxing and makes you sleepy and tranquil.

• A hot milky drink at bedtime will help you drop off, and you can also induce sleep by reading a calming book, listening to music or the radio.

• Deep breathing and relaxation exercises are excellent treatments for insomnia.

• Instead of worrying about your lack of sleep, get up and do something – perhaps a job that you've been putting off for some time.

• If you have worries that are stopping you from sleeping, to help clear your mind, visualize each one written on a piece of paper. Then mentally screw the paper up and throw it away.

REST AND RELAXATION

One of the aspects of later pregnancy that you may become concerned about is your comfort. As your abdomen gets larger, sitting or lying in your usual positions becomes uncomfortable. If you lie flat on your back, the weight of your growing baby presses down on the major blood vessels and nerves that lie against the spine, possibly causing numbness and tingling pain, and even dizziness and shortness of breath. Lying on your side may be an answer; or use pillows for support.

TENSE-AND-RELAX TECHNIQUE

A good way to relax your body is to use the tense-and-relax technique. This is a pleasant aid to relaxation during pregnancy, and useful preparation for labour, when it is a great help to be able to relax most of the muscles in your body, so that your uterus contracts without the rest of your body tensing.

Your partner can help by touching you where he can see you are tensing up: you respond to his touch by relaxing. It is best to practise this drill twice a day for 15–20 minutes if you can.

Find a comfortable position lying on your back propped up with cushions (see below). Close your eyes. Try to clear your mind of any anxieties by breathing in and out slowly and regularly and concentrating all your attention on your breathing. When your mind is relaxed and your breathing deep and regular, begin the tense-and-relax routine. Work through one side of your upper body, then the other, tensing and relaxing each muscle. Roll your knees outwards, tense and relax your buttocks, thighs, calves and feet. Finally, tense then relax the muscles of your face, eyes and forehead.

Resting on your back
If you can't rest lying on your side, prop yourself up with plenty of pillows.

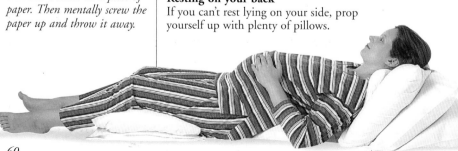

HEALTH PROBLEMS

Very few women go through pregnancy without suffering

from some complaint or ailment. These can be worrying,

but they are, in the main, uncomfortable rather than

serious. Most are caused by a combination of hormonal

changes and the extra weight that you have to carry and

can be treated fairly easily or else must be coped with

patiently – they usually disappear when your baby is born.

Understanding what causes the problem is half the battle

but, more importantly perhaps, it enables you to

differentiate between those problems that are just irritating

and those that are potentially serious.

COMMON COMPLAINTS

During pregnancy you may experience a number of discomforts that are often no more than irritating. Most are caused by a combination of hormonal changes and the extra strain that your body is experiencing; they can be treated very simply and are nothing to worry about. A few, however, can be serious, so be aware of the symptoms and be prepared to act promptly if you

COMPLAINT	WHY IT HAPPENS
Backache is usually a general discomfort across the lower part of the back, often with pain across the buttocks and down the legs. It can occur when you have been standing for too long with bad posture or after lifting a heavy weight, especially during the third trimester.	High progesterone levels cause softening and stretching of the ligaments of the pelvic bones, allowing the baby to be born. The ligaments of the spine also relax, putting extra strain on the joints of the back and hips.
Intensely painful low backache may also occur when you rotate your spine and pelvis in opposite directions, such as when you turn over sideways in bed.	The baby is resting against your sacroiliac joint, which is located some 7.5cm (3in) in from the top of your buttocks. Rotary movements of the spine and pelvis open and close the sacroiliac joint, causing pain.
Carpal tunnel syndrome is a sensation of pins and needles, mainly in the thumb and first finger, with numbness and sometimes weakness. Occasionally the whole hand and forearm are affected. It can occur from conception onwards.	Pressure on the nerve that passes from the arm to the hand along the front of the wrist. The pressure is caused by swelling of the carpal tunnel (a ring of fibres around the wrist under which the nerve passes) owing to water retention.
Constipation is when you have dry, hard stools that are difficult to pass. It can occur from conception onwards.	Progesterone relaxes the muscles in the intestinal walls, so there are fewer contractions to push the food along. Consequently much more water than usual is absorbed from the stool in the colon, making it hard and dry. Stools may be less frequent, too.
Cramp is a sudden pain in the thigh, calf and/or foot, followed by a general ache that lasts for some time. It tends to be more common in the third trimester, and usually wakes you from sleep.	Cramp is thought to be caused by low calcium levels in the blood, or it may be due to salt deficiency. Check with your doctor.

suspect all may not be well. Vaginal bleeding at any stage of pregnancy, for example, should always be taken seriously. It may indicate an abnormally placed placenta, placenta praevia (see p. 70), or it may be a warning of imminent miscarriage. Both of these conditions require prompt medical treatment.

If you have a pre-existing medical condition, such as diabetes or AIDS, you will need special monitoring and advice throughout your pregnancy.

WHAT CAN BE DONE

Massage may help (see p. 40). Do exercises to strengthen your spine. Make sure your mattress is firm. Lift heavy weights correctly. Try to improve your posture and avoid high-heeled shoes. If the pain runs down your leg towards your foot, consult your doctor in case it's a slipped disc.

Osteopathic manipulation can help you in even the most severe cases. Backache usually eases by itself in the fifth month when the fetus tips forward – although you may not want to wait that long! If it does not ease, consult a physiotherapist – you may need to wear a support belt.

Diuretics prescribed by your doctor may alleviate the symptoms. A splint on the wrist at night may help, as may holding your hand above your head and wiggling your fingers. Acupuncture may help. Sleep with your arm on a pillow. Symptoms usually disappear soon after delivery.

Drink lots of water. Eat as much roughage in the form of fruit, vegetables, and fibre as you can. Walk briskly for at least 20 minutes a day. Don't take a laxative without consulting your doctor. Natural fibre laxatives are best as they simply increase the amount of water in the stool, making it soft. Figs and prunes will also do the job.

Massage the area very firmly. Flex your foot up and push into the heel. You may be prescribed calcium or salt tablets if your levels are low, but don't self-prescribe without first consulting your doctor. Avoid pointing your toes.

RISK TO BABY

None.

None.

None.

None.

Relieving cramp
Keeping your foot flexed, make circling movements with your lower leg, first in one direction, then the other.

63

COMMON COMPLAINTS (CONTINUED)

COMPLAINT	WHY IT HAPPENS
Diarrhoea is when you have soft, watery stools, requiring frequent visits to the toilet. It can occur at any time.	Usually because an infection by bacteria or a virus is present.
Faintness is a feeling of dizziness or vertigo that occurs suddenly, making you unsteady on your feet. It can come on if you stand up too quickly, or have been on your feet for too long, especially in hot weather.	A lack of blood supply to the brain, often caused by pooling of the blood in the legs and feet when standing, together with the demands of the uterus for an increased blood supply.

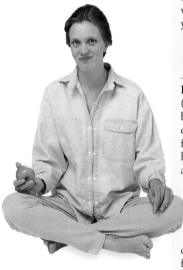

Coping with faintness
If you do feel faint, put your head as far down as you can – between your knees if you can still manage it! When you feel better, get up slowly.

Heartburn is a burning sensation just behind the breastbone, sometimes with regurgitation of stomach acid into the mouth. It happens most commonly on lying down, coughing, straining when passing a stool, and when you are lifting heavy weights.	Early in pregnancy, the muscular valve at the entrance to the stomach relaxes under the influence of progesterone. This allows stomach acid to flow up into the oesophagus, causing a burning sensation. Later in pregnancy, the baby can press up on the stomach, forcing the contents back into the oesophagus.
High blood pressure (hypertension) is an increase in blood pressure. It can be mild or severe, and there may be no, few, or some symptoms such as headaches, visual disturbances, and vomiting. Water retention with swelling of the feet, hands and ankles may also occur. It can happen at any time, but it is more likely to occur near term. It is more common in women having their first baby, especially if they are over 35, and also in women having more than one baby. It is important because it may herald pre-eclampsia (see p. 70).	The cause is not fully understood. In some women, cells from the placenta produce chemicals called vasoconstrictors that may cause the blood vessels to constrict. This may cause the blood pressure to rise, and the kidneys to retain sodium, leading to water retention.

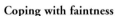

Avoiding heartburn
To prevent your stomach becoming overfull, eat smaller meals. Learn to snack on nutritious food and split large meals if they fill you up.

WHAT CAN BE DONE

RISK TO BABY

Increase your water intake to 12–14 glasses a day to replace lost fluid. This will ensure that your blood pressure remains normal. Consult your doctor, who will test your stools for infection and give you the appropriate treatment.

Diarrhoea can cause dehydration and loss of calories that can put your baby at risk if it goes untreated for a long time. If it is profuse and protracted, you will need to be hospitalized for intravenous feeding.

Avoid standing for long periods. Always sit or lie down when you feel dizzy. Don't get up suddenly from sitting or get out of a hot bath too quickly. Keep cool in hot weather. If dizzy, sit with your head between knees – if you still can – or lie down with your feet higher than your head.

None, unless you fall very heavily on to your stomach.

Keep meals small so that the stomach is never overfilled. Sleep propped up with several pillows. A glass of milk at bedtime will help to neutralize stomach acid. Your doctor may prescribe antacids, but only in the later stages of pregnancy.

None.

If you suffered from high blood pressure before you were pregnant, tell your doctor. Keep an eye on your weight. Always report persistent headaches and nausea.

Your doctor will test your blood pressure and urine, and look for any swelling (see p. 68) of your hands, face and ankles at each antenatal visit. He or she will almost certainly increase the frequency of your antenatal visits.

If your blood pressure goes up at any stage of your pregnancy, you will be advised to stay in bed and rest, and your doctor will suggest home visits.

If the rise is severe, you will be admitted to hospital, where you can be monitored continuously. If the baby appears to be suffering, labour may be induced or you may have a Caesarean section. Your blood pressure will return to normal once your baby has been born.

Pregnancy-induced hypertension or pre-eclampsia (see p. 70), can slow the baby's growth rate, owing to a reduced blood flow to the uterus. The baby may also be short of oxygen. Both these factors may lead to low birthweight. There is a severe form called eclampsia, which is life-threatening. Fortunately this is now very rare in the West, owing to excellent antenatal care that spots the signs at a very early stage.

COMMON COMPLAINTS (CONTINUED)

COMPLAINT	WHY IT HAPPENS
Insomnia is the inability to sleep at night, which makes you tired and irritable during the day. It can happen at any time from conception onwards.	Your baby lives on a 24-hour clock with a metabolism that keeps going even when you want to sleep. This can affect your body's responses. Other causes include night sweats, a need to empty your bladder more frequently, particularly during the third trimester, and difficulty in getting comfortable.
Mood swings describes rapid, uncharacteristic changes in mood, often with unexplained crying and anxiety attacks. They are common from conception onwards, but are especially likely to occur in the third trimester.	Changes in your hormone balance during pregnancy have a depressant effect on the nervous system, causing symptoms similar to those that can occur pre-menstrually. A change to your self-image and a possible identity crisis may also have profound effects as your pregnancy progresses. Mixed feelings about your pregnancy and parenthood can cause sudden shifts in your moods.
Morning sickness is a feeling of nausea, sometimes with vomiting. Contrary to its name, it can occur at any time of the day, but generally it happens when you haven't eaten, or after a long night's sleep. These symptoms often occur in the first trimester, but they usually ease off later on.	The main cause is low blood sugar, but pregnancy hormones may irritate the stomach directly.
Piles are dilated veins in the rectum (for varicose veins – see p. 68) that may protrude from the anus. Usually they do not occur until the second trimester.	Your increasingly larger baby presses down on your rectum and impedes blood flow to the heart. The blood therefore pools, causing the veins to dilate to accommodate the dammed-up blood.

Self-massage
Massaging your face, temples and neck is an effective way of relieving tension and may help dispel insomnia.

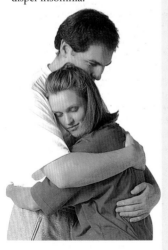

Coping with mood swings
A reassuring cuddle is probably just what you need when you're feeling anxious and upset.

WHAT CAN BE DONE

A warm bath and a hot milky drink may help, as may a relaxing massage (see p. 40). Watch television or read until you feel tired and sleepy. Find a comfortable position, and try to stay cool. Your doctor will not prescribe sleeping pills until the third trimester, and then only if you are exhausted by lack of sleep, because they can cross the placenta and affect the baby.

As long as depression doesn't become the dominant mood, you should consider these feelings as natural. Temporary depression, anxiety and confusion can occur even in the easiest of pregnancies. Talk to your partner about your worries and if you cannot cope, talk to your doctor. (See also p. 42.)

Some food will provide relief from nausea, so eat little and often. Eat high-carbohydrate foods such as bread, pasta, potatoes, rice and cereals, which provide long-lasting energy. Avoid fatty foods and coffee, which can trigger nausea, as can the smell of frying food, cigarette smoke and other strong smells.

Glucose sweets or drinks can help, so keep some in your car, desk or handbag. To prevent morning sickness first thing, put a glass of water and a plain biscuit or two by your bed before sleeping, and have them 15 minutes before you get out of bed.

Drink extra fluids such as fruit juice or skimmed milk – if you can keep them down.

Keep your bowels regular and the stools soft by eating sufficient fibre – this will help you avoid straining. Don't lift weights, because this increases intra-abdominal pressure and back pressure in the rectal veins. Have coughs treated promptly for the same reasons. Aromatherapy may be able to relieve symptoms.

RISK TO BABY

None.

None.

In its severe form (called hyperemesis gravidarum), excessive vomiting can deplete your fluid and mineral levels, leading to low blood pressure. This is always harmful to your baby. Inform your doctor if you vomit more than three times a day for three days. In very severe cases, hospitalization may be necessary to replace the fluids that you have lost.

None.

COMMON COMPLAINTS (CONTINUED)

COMPLAINT	WHY IT HAPPENS
Rib pain can be felt as extreme soreness and tenderness of the ribs, usually on the right side, just below the breasts. The pain is more severe when sitting down. It tends to occur mainly during the third trimester.	It is caused by pressure on the ribs as the baby grows in the abdomen. In addition, the baby can bruise your lower ribs with his or her head, or by excessive punching and kicking.
Tender painful breasts, with a feeling of heaviness and discomfort, and a tingling in the nipples, can be one of the first signs of pregnancy. It is present throughout, but usually increases towards term.	Hormones are preparing your breasts for lactation. The milk ducts are growing and being stretched as they fill with milk.
Thrush is a thick, white, curdy discharge from the vagina accompanied by dryness and intense itching around your vagina, vulva, perineum and, sometimes, your anus. You may also have pain when passing urine.	Thrush is an infection by the yeast *Candida albicans*, which occurs normally in the bowel. Infection occurs when the yeast grows uncontrolled by other bacteria, perhaps following a course of antibiotics. Thrush can happen at any time but it is particularly common in pregnancy. Excess sugar intake often aggravates it.
Varicose veins are swollen veins just below the skin. Although most common in the legs or anus, they can also occur in the vulva.	See also piles (p. 66)
Water retention happens when there is an increase in the amount of fluid present in the tissues. This causes swelling (oedema), especially of the ankles, feet, face and hands. Remove your rings before they become too tight.	Standing all day, especially in hot weather, can cause fluid to pool in the ankles and feet. High blood pressure (see p. 64), which is often associated with pregnancy, can force fluid from the bloodstream into the tissues, causing swelling and puffiness. The pregnancy hormones can cause retention of sodium by the kidneys, which in turn causes the body to retain fluid.

Wear comfortable clothes
Loose-fitting, comfortable clothing is essential during pregnancy. Tight-fitting tops will constrict you.

WHAT CAN BE DONE

RISK TO BABY

Wear loose clothes that won't restrict your ribs. Improve your posture – try not to slump forwards when sitting. Prop yourself up on cushions when you lie down. The pain eases when the baby's head drops into the pelvic cavity prior to birth.

None.

Wear a good supportive bra from early in pregnancy. If your breasts become very large, wear a bra at night as well (see p. 53). To prevent soreness, wash your breasts gently once a day with a mild soap and pat dry. Apply baby lotion or oil to your nipples if they become dry and sore.

None.

Avoid wearing tight underwear and trousers, as this encourages infection. Choose cotton underwear instead of man-made fibres. The doctor will prescribe pessaries that you should place in your vagina at night, as directed. You will also be prescribed a cream that should be gently rubbed into the skin surrounding the vaginal opening and the anus. These treatments should stop the discharge and thus the itching.

The baby can become infected as he passes down the birth canal on delivery. If this happens, white clumps like curds of milk will appear in the baby's mouth. The baby must be treated promptly with a course of antifungal agents, which will quickly clear up the infection.

Avoid standing for long periods. Put your feet up whenever you can. Wear pregnancy support tights. Gentle massage of the legs may help prevent varicose veins, but do not massage the area if you have developed them.

None.

Avoid standing for prolonged periods. Whenever possible put your feet up. Avoid eating salty foods. Your doctor will check your hands, face and ankles for any swelling at each antenatal visit, and occasionally diuretics may be prescribed.

In extreme forms this is potentially dangerous – see pre-eclampsia, p. 70.

VAGINAL BLEEDING

Vaginal bleeding at any stage of pregnancy should be taken seriously. It may indicate an abnormally placed placenta, placenta praevia (see right), or it may be a warning of imminent miscarriage. Both of these conditions require prompt medical treatment.

However, vaginal bleeding occurs in the first trimester in about a quarter of all pregnancies. Over half of these continue, with delivery of a healthy baby at term.

If at any time during your pregnancy vaginal bleeding occurs, you should call your doctor and go to bed.

PRE-ECLAMPSIA

An illness unique to pregnancy, this may occur in as many as one in ten pregnancies and affects both mother and baby. It occurs most often in a first pregnancy or in multiple births, usually in the second half of pregnancy. The exact cause is unknown, although the risk is greatest if there's a family history.

It is potentially dangerous for the baby because the placenta becomes deficient and raises the mother's blood pressure, both of which can happen silently – often the first sign is swelling of the ankles, face and fingers. Another sign is protein in the urine. Untreated, the condition can progress to coma, fits and threat to the baby's life. Delivery is the only treatment.

MEDICAL CONDITIONS

The vast majority of pregnancies proceed to term without problems or emergencies. However, there are certain medical conditions that require treatment or careful antenatal monitoring.

Placenta praevia This is the medical term for the condition when the placenta is positioned "ahead of" the baby in the uterus. During labour it could prevent the baby's head from descending, or even if the placenta is not blocking the way, it could become dislodged and bleed. If placenta praevia is suspected, you'll have an ultrasound scan early on and if confirmed, at term, or even slightly earlier (37 weeks), your baby will be delivered by Caesarean section.

Diabetes Diabetic mothers deliver normal, healthy babies all the time so, of itself, diabetes, as long as it is well controlled through your pregnancy, poses no threat to you or your baby. If you're an established diabetic, you'll be monitored closely throughout pregnancy and your dose of insulin may be adjusted.

Pregnancy can "unmask" a tendency to develop gestational diabetes, which can be controlled through diet, and which normally disappears after delivery. Babies of diabetic mothers can grow very large and if yours does, you may be induced before term so that he can still be born vaginally. At antenatal visits, your blood sugar, blood pressure and urine are checked and your diet carefully monitored.

HIV Being HIV positive shouldn't affect your pregnancy, nor will pregnancy necessarily precipitate AIDS in yourself. Pregnancy, however, does alter your immune state and you're less able to fight infections. You must take care of yourself in terms of eating well, staying fit and getting enough rest. Nowadays, you'll be given special care and will probably have several specialists as well as your midwife caring for you. Your condition can remain confidential.

Your baby is at risk – you have a one in five chance of passing on HIV to your baby in the womb. Delivery by Caesarean section and taking the drug AZT reduce this chance. You should also avoid breastfeeding.

A SENSUAL PREGNANCY

A woman undergoes many physical, emotional and
psychological changes during pregnancy, which can
influence her attitude to and enjoyment of sex. The high
levels of female hormones present in the body during
pregnancy may mean that you have the potential to enjoy
all levels of physical closeness with your partner far more
than ever before. However, because of any physical
discomforts such as nausea and fatigue, you may feel less
interested in sex. This can easily influence other aspects of
your relationship. Such problems can often be averted or
resolved by letting your partner know how you feel.

YOUR HORMONES

A woman undergoes many physical, emotional and psychological changes during pregnancy, which will influence her attitude to sex and her enjoyment of it. These changes are due mainly to the vastly increased levels of hormones circulating in her body.

The most important hormones involved in maintaining pregnancy are progesterone and oestrogen. In the early days of a pregnancy these are produced by the corpus luteum *in the ovary. However, once the embryo has implanted in the womb lining, it and the developing placenta take over as the primary sources of progesterone and oestrogen.*

The increase in the amounts of progesterone and oestrogen circulating in the body is swift and dramatic. The level of progesterone rises to ten times what it was before conception, while the amount of oestrogen produced in a single day is equivalent to that generated by a non-pregnant woman's ovaries in three years. In fact, during the course of a single pregnancy, a woman will produce as much oestrogen as a non-pregnant woman could in 150 years.

Progesterone and oestrogen induce a sense of well-being and also lead to shining hair, supple and glowing skin, and an aura of tranquillity and contentment.

ENHANCED SENSUALITY

Unless there are medical reasons for abstaining, sexual intercourse is safe and permissible during pregnancy. Moreover, every pregnant woman has the potential to enjoy sex possibly more than she ever has before.

The desire for sex and the enjoyment of it varies widely, not only from one woman to another during pregnancy, but also in the same woman at different times throughout its duration. Typically, though, there is a decline in interest in sex during the first trimester (especially if you are suffering from tiredness and nausea), followed by an increase in the second trimester, and then another decline in the third trimester.

When a pregnant woman does have sex, she may find it far more exciting and satisfying than it was before she conceived. In fact, a woman will sometimes achieve orgasm or multiple orgasms for the first time when she is pregnant. This enhanced sexuality is principally because of the high levels of female hormones and pregnancy hormones that circulate throughout her body when she is pregnant (see column, left). These cause a number of important changes to her breasts and sexual organs, making them more sensitive and responsive.

EROTICISM DURING PREGNANCY

One of the effects of the rise in oestrogen levels during pregnancy is an increase in blood flow, especially in the pelvic area. Because of this, the vagina and its folds (the labia) become slightly stretched and swollen. This stretching and swelling, which normally occur only during sexual excitement, make the sensory nerve endings hypersensitive, resulting in rapid arousal.

The breasts start to enlarge almost as soon as pregnancy occurs and one of the classic signs of pregnancy is sensitive, enlarged breasts with nipples that may tingle or even feel painful. The increased sensitivity of the breasts makes them a focus of sensory arousal, and a woman can feel enhanced sensations when her nipples and breasts are caressed and kissed by her partner. This sexual foreplay can also result in the arousal of the clitoris and the vagina.

Because of the increased blood flow, the vaginal secretions are quite profuse, so a pregnant woman usually becomes ready for penetration much earlier than usual. Penetration is particularly easy because of this, and a climax can be achieved quite quickly if the clitoris is stimulated simultaneously. The intensity of orgasm may reach new heights and the time taken to "come down" from an orgasm can be greatly extended. This is evident in the labia minora and the lower end of the vagina, which can remain swollen for anything up to two hours after orgasm, particularly in the last trimester.

Incidental to stimulating the whole of the genital area, the pregnancy hormones stimulate the production of a hormone that results in deeper skin pigmentation – particularly in the nipple area. Darkening of the nipples can act as a sexual signal to a man, making his partner's breasts very attractive to him.

WHEN TO MAKE LOVE

You can make love whenever you want to, as long as it's not too athletic and there are no medical reasons for you to forego it. Good sex in pregnancy helps prepare you for childbirth by keeping your pelvic muscles strong and supple. As at any other time, it also bonds you closer to your partner, which will help you cope much better with the stresses of parenthood.

There is absolutely no physical reason why a woman having a normal pregnancy should not enjoy sexual relations with her partner to the full and, if both partners are willing, sex need not stop any earlier than the onset of labour. In a low-risk pregnancy, the uterine spasms that accompany orgasms are perfectly safe, and in late pregnancy may be beneficial because they help prepare the uterus for the rigours of labour.

It is a fallacy that sex can cause an infection during pregnancy and may harm the baby – infection is virtually impossible because the cervix is closed and has a tough mucus plug that prevents the ascent of bacteria into the uterus. In addition, the baby is completely enclosed within the amniotic sac, which resists rupture even when under great pressure and cushions him against all external forces (including the weight of a partner during intercourse).

It goes without saying, however, that extremely athletic sex is not a good idea, because it may cause soreness and abrasions and a pregnant woman should be free of these unnecessary discomforts.

BUILDING YOUR RELATIONSHIP

The physical and emotional changes that take place during pregnancy will inevitably have an impact on your sexual relationship with your partner. Love and understanding will help you to minimize any problems that may arise.

As pregnancy advances you may find that you have to change your sexual habits, and the best way to approach this change is to realize that it is an opportunity to build on and enhance the physical side of your relationship. For instance, it might prompt you to explore (perhaps for the first time) the pleasures of new lovemaking positions and of other forms of sexual activity such as mutual masturbation and oral sex.

Try to understand any changes in your own and your partner's sexual desires, and be open with each other when discussing your needs, but never allow your sex life to become the dominant feature of your overall relationship. Concentrate on loving rather than lovemaking, and if at any time you or your partner don't feel like sex, rediscover the intimacy and joy of simply being with the one you love.

YOUR PARTNER'S DO'S AND DON'TS

By making a few adjustments to your lovemaking you can make the experience happier for the mother-to-be.

Do:

• *Be tender, romantic, patient and understanding.*

• *Use different kinds of stroking, such as a firm hand over her abdomen if the baby is kicking.*

• *Keep your weight off her stomach and breasts when making love.*

• *Use lots of pillows for greater comfort and to get the right angles around the curves of her body.*

• *Take your time when lovemaking, and don't be afraid to experiment.*

Don't:

• *Force her to make love if she doesn't feel like it.*

• *Expect her to have simultaneous orgasms – or even one orgasm.*

MAKING LOVE

You can continue making love as late into pregnancy as you wish, as long as there are no medical reasons for abstaining from it (see p. 76). Your baby, safe within your uterus, cannot be harmed by any normal sexual activity, and probably enjoys sex as much as you do because your hormones reach him through the placenta.

In the early months you can use any lovemaking position you choose, but as your abdomen swells you will probably find that making love in some positions, particularly the missionary position, with your partner on top, becomes uncomfortable.

When this happens, there are plenty of other erotic and exciting positions to use. In addition, these alternatives are often the best positions to use when you first resume lovemaking after the birth of your baby.

WOMAN-ON-TOP POSITIONS

You will probably find these most comfortable from the second trimester onwards. As your abdomen enlarges, you can lift yourself further off his stomach by supporting yourself on your knees. In this way, you can avoid too much pressure on your abdomen and breasts. In these positions, too, you can better control the depth of your partner's penetration as well as the speed and rhythm of your lovemaking.

These positions allow a great deal of intimacy. You and your partner have your hands free to caress and stroke each other and he can easily reach your breasts with his mouth. Alternatively, you can brush his chest with your breasts to stimulate him further.

KNEELING AND SIDE-BY-SIDE POSITIONS

These positions, many of which involve entering from behind, are useful during pregnancy, particularly if you don't feel very comfortable lying flat on your back, or at those times when you do not want to take too active a part in the lovemaking.

Kneeling positions allow your partner much freedom of movement and let him vary the amount of penetration. Side-by-side positions are not only comfortable but permit plenty of passionate kissing and caressing. The "spoons" position, so called because the partners nestle together like a pair of spoons, will also be useful if you experience any soreness or discomfort when you resume lovemaking after you have given birth, especially if you have had a tear or an episiotomy.

A variation on this position, with the woman lying on her back on top of her partner, frees her from any pressure on her abdomen while her partner has complete access to her vagina. He can continue to stimulate her either with his hand or his penis.

SITTING POSITIONS

Most useful in the middle and late months, these positions don't allow a lot of movement but they are comfortable for both partners and alleviate pressure on the abdomen. In addition, the depth of penetration can be controlled. In these positions, your partner sits on a sturdy, comfortable chair or the edge of the bed and you sit on his lap, either facing him (if your abdomen is not too big), facing to one side, or facing away from him.

When you are facing to one side or away from your partner, he can use his hands to caress your body and breasts and to stimulate your clitoris. In addition, because his range of movement is limited, you have control of the sexual tempo.

ANXIETIES

Even without a pregnancy and the attendant physical and emotional adjustments you both need to make, everyone experiences difficulties in their love life from time to time. There's reason enough for any woman to feel weary in pregnancy; a disappearing waistline, sore breasts, abdominal discomfort, the need to empty the bladder frequently, all militate against passionate sex. The man (and sometimes both partners) may fear that sex can somehow harm the baby (it can't; if anything your baby enjoys it). Talking things over, however, is essential, not only to explore different options and find comfortable positions but also to discuss your feelings about the move from partnership into parenthood.

Loving touch
During pregnancy, when sex is not as easy or desirable as before, touching, kissing and cuddling is a way of maintaining the loving bonds between a couple.

75

WHEN SEX MAY BE INADVISABLE

In some high-risk pregnancies, intercourse must be avoided at certain times or sometimes completely.

Your doctor will warn you if there is any risk of sexual activity being a danger to your pregnancy, and advise you on what is safe – and when. You should always make sure that he or she explains the problem fully, so that you are completely clear about what you can and cannot safely do.

The most common reasons and times for restricting intercourse during pregnancy are:

• At any time if there is any sign of bleeding. The bleeding may well be quite harmless, but you should consult your doctor without delay.

• If you have a history of miscarriage in the first trimester or if you are showing signs that you might miscarry early in pregnancy.

• If placenta praevia is suspected or confirmed (see p. 70).

• In the last trimester if you have a multiple pregnancy.

• In the last 12 weeks if you have a history of premature labour or if you are showing signs that you might go into premature labour.

• If your waters have broken.

SEXUAL PROBLEMS

During pregnancy, there are numerous physical and emotional factors that can diminish your enjoyment of sex. Fortunately, the few that actually prevent you from having intercourse are relatively uncommon (see left).

LOWERED SEX DRIVE

Many women feel that their bodies become less and less attractive as pregnancy progresses and this lack of confidence about their appearance often leads to a lowered inclination for sex. It is also difficult to feel attractive and sexy if you're suffering from the nausea and extreme fatigue of early pregnancy. In the second trimester, once free of these distractions, most women find that their interest and pleasure in sex returns. Towards the end of pregnancy, though, libido may wane again, largely due once more to fatigue.

Hormone levels can swing quite violently during pregnancy and you may find that you're emotionally volatile, switching from contentment to sadness and tearfulness, and then to great elation. All of this is perfectly normal but, of course, it can have an adverse effect on your sexual relationship with your partner. If it does, you must be open with your partner and honest about your feelings – and if you don't want to make love because you feel physically ill or excessively tired, tell him why – otherwise he could easily feel responsible, or worse, that you're rejecting him.

DISCOMFORT

As pregnancy progresses, partly as a result of high oestrogen levels and partly due to fluid retention, your body becomes very sensitive to touch – especially the breasts, labia and outer part of the vagina. This can mean that you have a heightened sexual response (see p. 72) but sometimes this sensitivity can verge on tenderness and foreplay may be unpleasant. Your engorged genitals may become swollen and aching after orgasm and can remain so for some time; this can cause a feeling of unrelieved fullness, which may make sex less satisfying. The sexual positions you have enjoyed may become uncomfortable. A little experimentation with non-penetrative sex, mutual masturbation and new positions may be the answer.

USEFUL ADDRESSES

Active Birth Centre
Bickerton House,
25 Bickerton Road,
London N19 5JT
Tel: 0171 561 9006

Information and classes on active involvement in childbirth at home or in hospital

AIMS (Association for Improvements in Maternity Services)
40 Kingswood Avenue,
London NW6 6LS
Tel: 0181 960 5585

Pressure group for parents to have the maternity services they want

APEC (Action on Pre-eclampsia)
31–33 College Road,
Harrow, Middlesex HA1 1EJ
Tel: 01923 266778

Aqua Birth Pools
Active Birth Centre,
Bickerton House,
25 Bickerton Road,
London N19 5JT
Tel: 0171 561 9006

For the hire of a portable water birth pool

Association of Breastfeeding Mothers
PO Box 441, St Albans,
Herts AL4 0AS
Tel: 0181 778 4769

A 24-hour telephone service for mothers. Supplies network of breastfeeding counsellors

Birthworks
Unit 3F, Brent Mill Trading Estate, South Brent,
Devon TQ10 9YT
Tel: 01364 72802

Advice and literature on water births, birth pools for hire

British Acupuncture Council
Park House,
206–208 Latimer Road,
London W2 6RE
Tel: 0181 964 0222

British Diabetic Association
10 Queen Anne Street,
London W1M 0BD
Tel: 0171 323 1531

British Epilepsy Association
Anstey House,
40 Hanover Square,
Leeds LS3 1BE
Tel: 01132 439393

British Homeopathy Association
27a Devonshire Street,
London W1N 1RJ
Tel: 0171-935 2163

Caesarean Support Network
55 Cooil Drive,
Douglas, Isle of Man,
Tel: 01254 661269 (after 6 pm)

Down's Syndrome Association
155 Mitcham Road,
London SW17 9PG
Tel: 0181 682 4001

Advice on the care of children with Down's syndrome

Foresight
28 The Paddock, Godalming,
Surrey GU7 1XD
Tel: 01483 427839

Pre-pregnancy advice and consultation on infertility and miscarriage; send SAE

National Childbirth Trust
Alexandra House,
Oldham Terrace, Acton,
London W3 6NH
Tel: 0181 992 8637

Nationwide antenatal classes and practical postnatal help

RCOG (Royal College of Obstetricians and Gynaecologists)
27 Sussex Place, Regent's Park,
London NW1 4RG
Tel: 0171 262 5425

Helpline and leaflets

Royal College of Midwives
15 Mansfield Street,
London W1M 0BE
Tel: 0171 580 6523/4/5

St Mary's Hospital Recurrent Miscarriage Clinic
Winston Churchill Wing,
Praed Street,
London W2 1NY
Tel: 0171 258 0285

SANDS (Stillbirth and Neonatal Death Society)
28 Portland Place,
London W1N 4DE.
Tel: 0171 436 5881

National support network for bereaved parents

TAMBA (Twins and Multiple Birth Association)
PO Box 30, Little Sutton,
South Wirral L66 1TH
Tel: 0151 348 0020

Offers support before and after multiple births

Vegetarian Society
Parkdale, Dunham Road,
Altrincham,
Cheshire WA14 4QG
Tel: 0161 928 0793

Nutritional advice for pregnant women who are vegetarians

Women's Health
52 Featherstone Street,
London EC1Y 8RT
Tel: 0171 251 6580

Advice on reproductive health

INDEX

ACKNOWLEDGMENTS

Dorling Kindersley would like to thank the following individuals and organizations for their contributions to this book.

PHOTOGRAPHY
All photographs by Ranald Mackechnie except:
Hattie Young page 12.

MEDICAL CONSULTANTS
Gwen Atwood; Leonora Branski; Dr. Nigel Brown; Dr. Felicity Challoner; Prof. Geoffrey Chamberlain; The Hallam Medical Centre; Dr. Kypros Nicolaides; Prof. Cheryl Tickle; Dr. Robert Whittle.

EQUIPMENT
Mothercare UK Ltd – maternity and baby clothes; equipment; and toys.

INDEX
Hilary Bird

TEXT FILM OUTPUT
The Brightside Partnership, London